Study Skills
and Tomorrow's
Doctors

Cartoons by Jane Ancona

For WB Saunders Company Ltd

Publisher: Laurence Hunter
Project Editor: Jane Shanks
Copy Editor: Alison Gale
Project Controller: Nancy Arnott
Design: Erik Bigland

Study Skills and Tomorrow's Doctors

David W. Bullimore MD MRCP BSc DipMedEd

Consultant Physician and Gastroenterologist
Barnsley District General Hospital NHS Trust
South Yorkshire
UK

WB Saunders Company Ltd

Edinburgh London Philadelphia Toronto Sydney Tokyo 1998

WB Saunders Company Ltd   1–3 Baxter's Place
Leith Walk
Edinburgh EH1 3AF
24–28 Oval Road
London NW1 7DX

The Curtis Center
Independence Square West
Philadelphia, PA 19106-3399, USA

Harcourt Brace & Company
55 Horner Avenue
Toronto, Ontario M8Z 4X6, Canada

Harcourt Brace & Company, Australia
30-52 Smidmore Street
Marrickville, NSW 2204, Australia

Harcourt Brace & Company, Japan
Ichibancho Central Building, 22-1 Ichibancho
Chiyoda-ku, Tokyo 102, Japan

A catalogue record for this book is available from the British Library.

ISBN 0 7020 2287 X

Produced by Addison Wesley Longman China Limited, Hong Kong
EPC/01

Preface

Current medical courses are new, challenging and very different from those of ten or even five years ago. This book explains why these changes are taking place and what they are. It is also about the study skills which students need to cope with the modern medical course and which will equip them with the lifelong learning skills that they will need throughout their future career.

The advice given is based on long experience of educating students and on an appreciation that their individual needs differ. It has benefited from much frank feedback from current, past and intending students about their experience as learners! The book is therefore meant primarily for current medical students and for those applying for medical courses who wish to have a firm grasp of the likely nature of such courses. It is written in a style which I hope will provide both enlightenment and enjoyment, as it is my belief that the latter enhances the former.

I hope that many tutors and the parents (or other relatives) of students will also find the book of use and interest. Tutors should find it useful for its summary of the changes now taking place in medical courses and for its ideas on how students can be helped to learn. Parents of current and intending students should find it provides help in understanding the course of study that their off-spring are undertaking or wishing to undertake, as well as the reasons behind the teaching and learning methods used, which may be different from their own experience of higher education.

Those entering medical school are gifted and enthusiastic. This book is to help ensure that their enthusiasm remains and that they meet the challenges of the course, and so succeed in qualifying with the right knowledge, skills and attitudes to form a firm foundation to their chosen career.

David Bullimore
1998

This book is dedicated to Shelagh, Sharon and Michael.

Acknowledgements

My thanks to the following colleagues at the University of Leeds, with whom I have had many enjoyable and enlightening discussions about medical education: Margaret Le Beau, Andrew Hill, Deborah Murdoch-Eaton and Patsy Stark. My thanks also to the General Medical Council, which so willingly gave permission to quote from its material. Responsibility for the interpretation of all material, and any resulting misinterpretation, is of course entirely my own.

David Bullimore

Contents

1

Starting point...

You almost certainly already possess two of the things that you need to succeed in a medical course: ability and intent. This book is about two other things which you also need. These are good study skills and a knowledge of the structure of a modern medical course.

The advice given on study skills is practical, to help you organize your studies and get the most from things such as lectures, work in small groups and clinical work. I hope that you will find this advice enjoyable as well as useful. The discussion of the structure of medical courses is about the new influences and developments that are reshaping medical education in order to meet the needs of the 21st century. These changes mean that the course you will be taking will, in many respects, be very different from those taken by doctors who have already qualified, even if they qualified only 5 years ago. The discussion is not dry, distant and academic – it is about how these changes will affect you in your studies, and could help to determine what sort of doctor you will become.

You might say, reasonably, that you see the use of a book describing changes in medical education, but why one about study skills? After all, the chances are that you are a motivated, intelligent and determined student. You probably have achieved better than three A levels, at grade B, or the equivalent, or expect to get such grades. If entering medical school as a graduate, you will have a first or upper second class honours degree. What is more, I have never met you – so am I being presumptuous in offering advice?

I would, of course, suggest that I am not. Although we have not met, I have met and been involved in the education of literally thousands of medical students. Among those students I cannot recall one whose intellectual ability was in doubt. But there is a reason for a study skills guide, and the reason is simple – while the vast majority of students complete their course successfully, a few do fall by the wayside and considerably more stumble along the way at some time or another. One of the most common reasons is poor study techniques. We spend so much time learning 'things' that many of us never take time to think about how we can learn better. Think back to the thousands of hours you spent in school. Most people cannot recall having even a single lesson to discuss or think about how we learn. One part of this book is to help redress that balance. While study skills have relevance whenever you acquire them, if you do so before or near the start of your course they will be of extra value. Your approach will be better from day one. This book does not provide a magic formula for successful studying, because individuals differ in their approach, but read through and dip into the guide to avoid making mistakes already made by others. This will help you to learn better and faster.

Let us lay to rest at this early stage one of the apocryphal stories about medical schools in the UK. They do *not* admit too many students in the first year, and then fail a set percentage in order to trim the student body down to size for later parts of the course. All students can be accommodated right through the course. The only reasons for failure to progress are failure of exams, changes of mind about wanting to do medicine, or personal or health problems. Personal and health problems are of course treated sympathetically and, in suitable cases, time out can be arranged. Use this book and you will not be in the first category, those who fail their exams.

Arguably, the second purpose of this book, to discuss how medical courses are changing, would not have been necessary a few years ago. There was a slow evolution in medical education taking place, but the general structure of courses had remained the same for over half a century in many institutions. This changed with the publication in 1993 by the General Medical Council (GMC) of the document *Tomorrow's Doctors*. The GMC has, among its many functions, statutory responsibility for ensuring that the standard of medical education in medical schools in the UK is in all respects appropriate and adequate. The proposals in *Tomorrow's Doctors* were quite radical, and are leading to new and quite different systems of medical education. These will produce graduates who are both more similar and more diverse than previous graduates. This apparent paradox will be explained along with the discussion of *Tomorrow's Doctors* (see Chapters 3 and 4).

There are at least four other parallel changes taking place in higher education and medical education:

- move to self-directed learning
- advances in computing and technology

- move to early clinical contact
- development of clinical skills learning centres (CSLCs).

First, throughout higher education there is a move towards more student-centred and self-directed learning (SDL). More of what is learnt is to be decided by the student rather than by the teacher, and students are required to take more responsibility for managing their own learning. Second, advances in computing and other technologies mean that there are both new ways of delivering material and new material to deliver. For instance, is it any longer necessary to have all students learning the same topic at the same time if you switch from a lecture session to a computer-aided learning (CAL) package? Third, there is a move to earlier clinical contact and more work outside the major teaching hospitals. Fourth, and most recently, there is the development of clinical skills learning centres (CSLCs) in most UK medical schools. These are developing embryos which have the potential to transform large areas of medical education if appropriately nurtured and incorporated into the curriculum. They will be discussed later in some detail. The above four additional factors have combined to become a powerful force for change (Fig. 1.1).

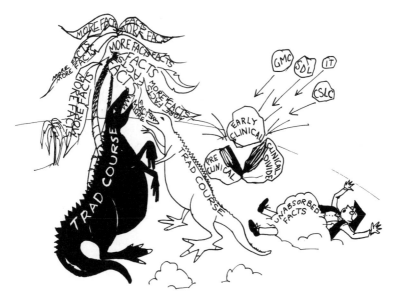

Fig. 1.1 Factual overload is only one of the pressures for change in the medical curriculum.

Medical courses in the UK consist of 5 or 6 years of undergraduate study plus a preregistration year, which is a year of supervised clinical experience. The quality of the preregistration experience is the responsibility of the university. Traditionally, the preregistration year has comprised 6 months' surgery and 6 months' medicine within a hospital, but this is now broadening, with the possibility of some work being in other specialties or outside the hospital sector. While this book is mainly about the undergraduate years, much is also applicable to the preregistration year and your future professional career.

Good luck with your studies. You are entering a rewarding, challenging and varied profession.

DIFFERENCES BETWEEN SCHOOL LIFE AND UNIVERSITY LIFE

While some of you will have had considerable and diverse experience between school and university, most of you and those fellow medics you see around you in Freshers' Week will be making a direct transition from school/college to university. Below we deal with some of the differences that you will meet. Those who do not make the transition directly fall into a number of groups, and we will also look at the advantages and disadvantages of being in one of these.

Some differences between school and university, such as size, are obvious but the differences are more than just ones of scale. One of the first things students find is that everyone else seems so bright. While they were near the very top of their form at school, now there are plenty of others who seem brighter. Don't panic. You have just moved up a few layers on life's intellectual pyramid. Nothing terrible has happened to you between school and university and you certainly have the ability to succeed on the course. On the plus side it means there are lots more interesting people to discuss medical (and non-medical) things with.

At school you are taught in relatively small groups of 30 or less by teachers whom you know and who know you. At university there will be some small group teaching but you will also be taught in large groups of 100 or more. In some universities, inter-departmental teaching to groups of 500 or more students takes place either in one large lecture auditorium or by remote video link between centres. You may never have seen the lecturer before and he/she may never lecture to you again. This can be daunting and disorientating at first. Take comfort – others will be feeling the same and you will soon get used to it.

School provides you with a framework of what you have to learn, whereas university gives you a lot more freedom to plan your work and decide when to do it. Indeed, it can be difficult to know just what it is you are supposed to know! Seek advice from tutors and other students. This increasing freedom, or requirement for you to direct, select and pursue your own studies, will be particularly marked in those medical schools which have moved furthest from offering traditional courses.

University life provides lots of attractions which compete with study. For many students it will be the first time that they have had to manage their own budget and live away from home. There are new friends to see, clubs of all sorts to join and many places to go for a night out. *So, an important message in this book is that of achieving the right balance between work and social life.* Those who work all the time are failing to develop themselves as individuals and missing much of what student life should offer. Those who play all the time will fail the course and themselves. You are at university to train to be an excellent doctor. It is a privilege. Get the balance right from early on, and don't fall behind because of lack of study.

STUDENT SUBGROUPS

While some problems are common to all students starting a new medical course, some are experienced by particular subgroups of students and can make them feel particularly vulnerable. In their turn, these students often have strengths, not fully appreciated by themselves, which enhance the life of the medical school and the quality of the course. So, it's worth considering the main subgroups, even if you are not a member of one, so that you can help them with their difficulties and benefit from their strengths:

- mature students
- recent graduates
- single parents
- 'gap' students
- non-UK students
- disabled students.

Mature students
By mature students I mean those who exceed the average age of the student body and who have been away from mainstream education for 5–8 years. Mature students in some disciplines can

be of virtually any age, but those in medical faculties rarely exceed 28–30 years of age at the time of entry. Some men or women will have spent several years starting to raise a family, others will have worked in the 'real world' and have varied experience. Examples I have known have practised in teaching, nursing, commerce or industry. All have had a first degree, but possibly no recent student experience. Common problems of mature students are that they feel they learn at a slower rate and remember less well than more recent students, and are less confident about the black-and-white nature of many decisions. From the tutor's point of view they are often welcome for their maturity, listening and organising skills, and their ability to put forward a balanced view – and also for their realization that few decisions in medicine are black-and-white.

Recent graduates

Problems faced by recent graduates are often related to the feeling of 'having to start all over again', especially if their original intention, as is the case for the majority, was to pursue a career in another discipline. There may be a good deal of repetition in the teaching of general skills and basic science early on from which they cannot gain exemption. This can lead to some frustration and boredom. For example, they may feel that the clinical lecturer talking about chest infections knows less bacteriology than they, as a graduate bacteriologist, do. (In all probability they are right. The technique is to listen to what else the clinician is saying about the presentation, management and prognosis of chest infections.) Graduates may already be in debt and are unlikely to have a grant to support them for their medical course. This puts them under even more financial pressure than the first-time undergraduate. However, they have many strengths apart from their subject-specific knowledge. They have a good honours degree, so have no doubts about their intellectual ability. They understand the academic processes of lectures, tutorials and practicals, and how libraries can best be used and databases searched. Equally importantly, they understand 'how student life works' and often their first degree course was at the same university, so they know their way around. They are valuable people to have in any student discussion group, academic or social.

Single parents

Being a single parent – male or female – is tough. Being a single parent and pursuing a medical course is extremely tough. It will continue to be so beyond graduation and into the first few years of professional life because of the unsocial and irregular hours of most junior hospital jobs. The successful will be both determined and organized, arranging for protected study time when they can usually work uninterrupted by their family (Fig. 1.2). The medical school will expect the single parent to fulfill the same course requirements as his or her colleagues, including periods of residency. The sensible student will of course check up on things such as the availability of crèche facilities at the university, if these will be required, and whether the medical school is prepared to review the location of residencies. For instance, if traditionally one of two attachments in a specialty is taken locally and the other in a far-flung hospital, the medical school might arrange two local attachments. Single parents often have broad experience to bring to the student body. They may have gone through the trauma of separation, divorce, the breakdown of a long-term relationship or the loss of a partner. They may have gone through the psychological trauma of an unplanned pregnancy and agonized over the decision as to whether to have an abortion or to keep the baby. All this experience allows them to give a different perspective to clinical problems and to the difficulties patients have in making medically 'clear-cut' decisions because of social and personal factors in their lives.

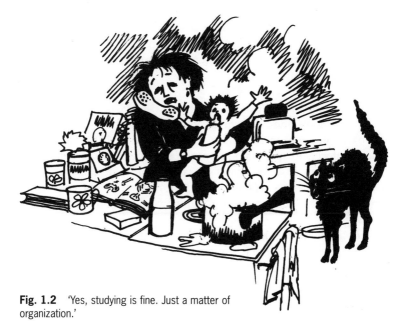

Fig. 1.2 'Yes, studying is fine. Just a matter of organization.'

One of the freedoms of university life is greater sexual freedom. An unplanned pregnancy during a university course is depressingly common and is often an emotional and academic disaster. Avoid it: the rule is simple, don't have unprotected intercourse even 'just this once'. Neither a full moon nor it being Freshers' Week provides contraceptive protection. Responsibility for avoiding unplanned pregnancy applies equally whether you are male or female, drunk or sober.

'Gap' students

It is becoming increasingly common for students to take a year off between school and university, although a slight wobble occurred in 1997/8 with the introduction of fees for study. Students can mature and change a lot during a year off, which is often spent travelling. There are two questions they must ask themselves when they return. The answer to both must be an unequivocal 'Yes'. One: 'Do I still want to train to be a doctor?'. Two: 'I know how to study. I have not studied for a year. Am I prepared to go back to several years of hard study?'. If the answers are 'Yes', gap students should have few additional problems arising from their year off, and socially have the advantage of a rich store of anecdotes – real, embellished and (frequently) imaginary. If the answer to either question is 'No' or 'Not really', decide before the course starts – not at the end of the first week, term or year. Remember that there are many other professions and occupations which are just as challenging and fulfilling as medicine. Changing your mind at this stage is wisdom not failure.

Students from outside the UK

Medical schools should have an individual member of staff who has particular responsibility for the welfare of overseas students. Check before you apply. The common attitude of 'I just treat them the same as the rest. You can't do fairer than that, can you?' fails to understand the particular difficulties of an overseas student trying to cope in a new country, in a new culture and in a foreign language.

Problems often relate to difficulties with both language and culture. How can you help yourself? Firstly, if your English is not fluent then sit near the front of the lecture theatre, where you can catch the eye of the lecturer. Sensitive lecturers will alter their pace of delivery, simplify the language of explanations and avoid colloquial phrases to help you – if they are aware that you are having difficulty keeping up. If you are sitting at the back of the lecture theatre your difficulty is less likely to be noticed. If you do not understand a phrase ask a fellow student, or the lecturer, at the end of the lecture. As an example, the colloquial phrase above, 'catch the eye of the lecturer', could easily be misunderstood. At other times, difficulties with language and differences in culture may combine to inhibit the overseas student. For example, a tutor may issue a challenging statement to his/her tutorial group to provoke discussion. A student who comes from an educational culture in which it is impolite to challenge the teacher may be left silent and feeling confused. If language fluency is also a concern of the student, he/she may be reluctant to speak. Such students may fail to realize that their colleagues do not mind giving them a little extra time or how envious most UK students are of their ability to speak a second language as well as most overseas students do.

Inevitably the cultural changes for a student coming to the UK for the first time from Iran or Kuwait are greater than those for a student from Switzerland or the Netherlands. But whichever country they are from, overseas students will be welcomed by the home students both for themselves and for the knowledge of different healthcare systems, cultural beliefs and values that they can bring into any discussion.

Disabled students

Many students with a disability will come direct from school or college. Depending on the nature of your disability you will have different requirements, and these need to be discussed early with the medical school and the university. Universities are large public organizations, which take willingly and seriously their responsibility for provision for students with a disability. For example, they may nominate specific individuals to help with problems such as wheelchair access or the difficulties faced by students with dyslexia. Enquire as appropriate. Most major lecture theatres have induction loops to aid those with hearing difficulties.

Occasionally students with general medical conditions, such as epilepsy or diabetes, are concerned about revealing this information when they apply to medical school. Please be reassured that it will not count against you in selection, but do tell us so that we can cope more easily should any problem arise. I once found my house officer unconscious and smelling of beer. Not knowing he was a diabetic wasted some valuable time in diagnosing his hypogly-caemic coma. His atypical stroppy behaviour earlier that evening was one of the clues (you rarely get audibly sworn at by your house officer – more usually, I suspect, it is sotto voce), as was his cold and clammy state while comatose.

Universities can help in many ways but cannot alter the geography of the town in which they are situated. If you suffer from cystic fibrosis or a heart condition and get short of breath on minor exertion, you should logically choose to study at a medical school in one of the less hilly reaches of the United Kingdom. Consider the geography when you apply. There is little point in being accepted in a city in which you cannot happily cope.

The strengths of students with disability, in terms of the experience and 'consumer viewpoint' that they bring, are self-evident. So is the realization they bring to other students that individuals are not defined by their disability but that the disability is just one component of their being.

HELP!

> '*I was much further out than you thought*
> *And not waving but drowning.*'
> (Stevie Smith, 1902–71)

It's a new life, with new excitement and, unfortunately, sometimes new problems. This can be the case whether you are a mainstream student or from a minority group. How do you get help if you run into difficulties, either personal or related to study?

The first thing to realize is that the best time to get help is early on, when a problem starts and before it gets too bad. The second is that asking for help will not be seen as a sign of weakness but of common sense. Who you will ask for help will depend on the problem and your preference. If you are having problems with a particular subject, then talk to a member of the staff whom you know within that department. Alternatively, or if your academic problems are more general, make an appointment to talk things over with the Academic Sub-Dean (or equivalent – the Undergraduate Office will advise). If there is a member of staff whom you feel is approachable you can arrange to see them, even if the specific area causing problems is not related to their course. Problems may be personal, emotional or financial rather than academic, and again the Academic Sub-Dean will be willing to give help and advice. An informal chat with friends or a phone call home might also give a silver lining to some of the clouds.

You should register with the Student Health Service or one of the local GPs when you arrive at medical school. Please do not wait to become ill before registering. Both provide the same wide range of services, and the same high degree of confidentiality, as your GP at home. The Welfare Office in the Students' Union will have a list of GPs who are able to take students onto their lists. The Welfare Office will also have a wide range of leaflets on many matters such as health, finances and housing, in addition to being available for confidential discussion. Many universities run a Nightline (or equivalent). This is a telephone service which students can use to discuss in confidence absolutely anything which is worrying them. Nightlines provide both an information service and a listening service. They are often run by sympathetic students, but remember that they are not professional counsellors. Professional confidential counselling is usually available through a Student Counselling Service. The Samaritans can also provide help and support. One common problem is wanting to make an appointment but not having the right telephone number, so in Box 1.1 below are a few contact suggestions and some blank slots for you to add your own. The important thing to understand is that any problem is best discussed early, and no matter how terrible the situation seems to be to you there is someone available who will spend time to find out how you can be helped.

Box 1.1 Contact numbers	
Student Counselling Service	☎
Welfare Office (Students' Union)	☎
Student Health Service	☎
General practitioner	☎
Personal tutor	☎
Academic tutor	☎
Samaritans (local number)	☎
Samaritans (national number)	☎ 0345 909090
	☎
	☎
	☎
	☎

2

Why medical courses needed changing

This is best understood in general terms by looking at a traditional medical course. While these varied, an account of my own experience has a generality of truth which I suspect holds across many medical schools.

A MEDICAL COURSE OF 20–25 YEARS AGO (through rose-tinted glasses)

Twenty to twenty five years ago the basic medical course was so well established in type that in many medical schools it changed little until recently. Entry requirements were three A levels at grade C or better, generally in chemistry, physics and biology (or maths). The course was in two parts – 2 years preclinical and 3 years clinical. The preclinical course provided the solid scientific basis for the clinical work: anatomy, physiology and biochemistry were studied in the first year, supplemented by pathology, microbiology and pharmacology in the second. The week consisted of 2 days of lectures plus 3 days of tutorials and practical work, detailed anatomical dissection of a cadaver forming the major part of the latter. Live patients were kept out of sight. Exams marked the completion of this first phase.

At this stage, a number of students opted to do an extra year's study in order to obtain a BSc honours degree in one of the preclinical subjects. The extra year was willingly funded in terms of maintenance grant and tuition fees by the local education authority. Students who took the BSc option were either neophytic academics or those who realized that in no other way could you get an honours degree for only 26 weeks' work, with the bonus of an additional long vacation thrown in. Dishonourably, I fell into the latter category.

Clinical studies consisted of attachments to a series of clinical firms in different specialties, starting with 3 months in each of medicine and surgery. You clerked, formed management plans and followed the (often prolonged) clinical stay of the six to twelve patients allocated to your care. The week was punctuated by two afternoons of lectures, teaching ward rounds and tutorials. Lecture afternoons were either three separate 1-hour lectures or the new 'integrated systems teaching'. For instance, in a session dealing with tuberculosis different aspects would be presented by clinician, microbiologist, pharmacologist, epidemiologist and radiologist. Anatomist, physiologist or biochemist was rarely involved, just as clinicians had not been seen during their courses. Teaching ward rounds were spent with 10–15 students standing around a hospital bed containing a 'case', which was presented by one student and then discussed by the group. Woe betide any student who had not fully clerked an allocated patient who had been in hospital for 24 hours or more or who had not seen their patient for follow-up during the previous 24 hours. Students came in to the hospital at 8.00 a.m. on rota to take blood samples before the 9.00 a.m. ward round. Evening surgical ward rounds, to see acute surgical cases admitted during the day before they went to surgery, were voluntary. Since teaching was excellent and you had the opportunity to make a diagnosis before the defining surgical incision, 10–12 of the 15-strong firm attended. Whatever time the evening ward rounds started, they finished at 10.00 p.m. so we could go to the pub afterwards.

We were warned by many in the university teaching hospitals that during our attachments in peripheral hospitals we would meet primitive conditions, and consultants who were frequently out of date and not fired by being in the heady atmosphere of constant academic research. We were delighted at the welcome we received in these hospitals, our incorporation as valued members of the team, the wide range of cases seen and often the astuteness and humanity of the clinicians who looked after us and the patients.

We were likewise warned that general practice was for the second-rate. This advice was ignored by several of the brightest in our year, who paused to intercalate and collect a first class honours degree, then registered and entered general practice with the minimum possible delay. Exposure to general practice was for 4 weeks. Two weeks were spent in an inner city practice, where I learnt that gas mantles were still used for lighting and that real poverty and malnutrition existed in Britain and affected health. Two more weeks were spent in a non-city practice. The Scilly Isles are very beautiful in April. The academic who organized the student–GP links provided himself with occasional amusement by playing word games. Thus, student 'Plumb' would be linked with GP 'Duff' to generate the name of the pudding, 'plum duff'. Such triviality was no hindrance to future greatness, and he subsequently rose to be chairman of the BMA.

Finals were a traditional combination of long and short cases plus written papers. There was also a viva, at which the examiner demonstrated his specialist knowledge and we our generalist ignorance.

House jobs started on August 1st with no induction and a one-in-two rota of 120 hours/week. There was no concept of overtime and therefore no overtime payment. You were part of a firm of two house officers, one registrar (or senior house officer, SHO) and two consultants. Sometimes there was also a senior registrar. Nursing staff were a combination of trained staff and trainees undergoing apprenticeship-style training. They were led by a sister or senior staff nurse, who always knew everything that was going on and provided guidance, support and the occasional night-time omelette to new house staff. Pressure on beds being less than now meant that on occasion a bed in a ward side-room provided overnight sanctuary for a post-party student or house officer unable to make it home. However, the lipstick, applied or transmitted, and inappro-priateness of attire was often a give-away the next morning. The long hours, the clinical firm structure, the nursing structure and having patients concentrated on two adjacent wards meant that you all knew each other well and good communication was informal and easy. House staff attended postgraduate meetings, but there was no formal house officer teaching or mentoring system – you learnt by observation and osmosis. The house officer year was considered your first year of employment, not your final year as a student.

You were paid around £1300/year – a considerable step up from the student grant of under £500/year. A shared flat cost £2–3/week and beer in the Students' Union was the equivalent of 10p/pint. The local rough cider was cheaper. It could be sweetened with a squeeze of lemon juice and also used as a dip to remove tarnish from metal objects (Fig. 2.1). Five students, two of whom were on army scholarships, had cars. The student body was generally left-wing, supported the Labour party (at a time when Labour was a left-wing party) and demonstrated about low grants and social injustice. We were condemned as being scruffy and lazy and told that we neither worked as hard nor were as intelligent and curious as our predecessors.

They were happy days.

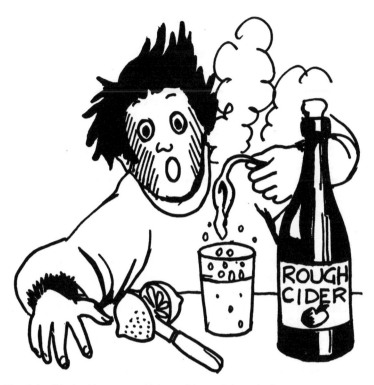

Fig. 2.1 'No, I said sweeten with lemon juice and *then* stir...'

A MEDICAL COURSE OF 20–25 YEARS AGO (the other reality)

Much preclinical teaching was to a level of detail not needed by a medical graduate and the volume overload was immense, especially in anatomy. Much was irrelevant. I have never used my detailed knowledge of mechanisms of photosynthesis, nor that of the metabolic pathways of nitrogen-fixing bacteria. The separation and dissociation of preclinical and clinical work meant knowledge was learnt without any useful applied context and frequently forgotten the moment that we walked out of the examination hall. We had come to be doctors but did not see any patients for 2 years. It was dispiriting and demotivating.

The clinical curriculum was undefined in scope and overloaded as a consequence by enthusiastic subspecialists. Teaching was opportunistic, utilizing whatever happened to be on the ward that day, and therefore patchy and frequently repetitive. Teachers varied, from the concerned and kind with high expectations of the students to the arrogant and bullying who enjoyed exercising their power. We did not know what we had to learn.

There was insufficient regard for the emotional, social and cultural needs of patients and the impact of their disease upon them. There was little idea that hospital care was but a minor component of a healthcare system which had to be integrated and used appropriately to deliver quality, economic health care where it was most needed. The view was rather that hospitals, especially teaching hospitals, were at the summit of a healthcare pyramid with a right to have first call on any resources. Scant regard was paid to learning about general practice or other community health services.

The house year was met unprepared and the workload and working hours were barbaric. Routine repetitive tasks and fatigue from the long hours prevented reflection and learning. The year was generally survivable if you were in a good working team of clinicians and nurses. For others it led to mental breakdown, marital breakdown and, on occasion, suicide.

For all the above reasons, the publication of *Tomorrow's Doctors* as a new framework for medical education which would overcome many of the existing problems of the traditional medical course was welcomed by medical schools and those who taught in them.

3
Tomorrow's Doctors: a first look

Tomorrow's Doctors was published by the General Medical Council (GMC) in December 1993. Its fuller title, *Tomorrow's Doctors. Recommendations on Undergraduate Medical Education,* better indicates its scope.

Since these recommendations will almost certainly form the framework of your medical course, we will look at the background to the publication and at some of its content in some detail. The Medical Education Committee of the GMC set out to produce *Tomorrow's Doctors* against a background of prolonged and accelerating change in medical care, from the viewpoints of scientific and technical advances and changes in the way that health care was being delivered in the community. Factors for change included external factors and others inherent in the educational process itself.

External factors were numerous:

1. The need to reinstate public health medicine and the epidemiology of disease. This had almost been dropped from many medical courses. With the resurgence of infectious diseases such as HIV and new-variant CJD, and a new emphasis on preventative medicine, such as the control of high blood lipid levels, it assumed a new importance.
2. The shift of balance as to where health care was taking place, with a move from hospital-based care to care in general practice for many diseases.
3. A greater sharing of care across professions and within multiprofessional teams.
4. An ageing, multiracial population with changing health needs.
5. New sciences (e.g. molecular medicine) and techniques (e.g. minimally invasive surgery).
6. Increased public expectations for health and the amelioration of disease.

7. The need for more extensive and improved doctor–patient communication, with the responsibility for decisions about treatment being taken by the patient, after informed discussion, rather than by the doctor.

Important though these changes were, the GMC considered that there were inherent factors which called for change even more pressingly and urgently. Were these inherent factors new? Indeed they were not, as quotations in *Tomorrow's Doctors* show:

- GMC, 1863: '…tendency to an overloading of the curriculum of education…followed by results injurious to the student.'
- GMC, 1869: 'Whoever will consider the great extent of the sciences which lies at the foundation of medicine and surgery will see that some limit must be assigned to the assessment of knowledge which can be fitly exacted.'
- Thomas Huxley, 1876: 'The burden we place on the medical students is far too heavy and it takes some doing to keep from breaking the intellectual back. A system of medical education that is actually calculated to obstruct the acquisition of sound knowledge and to heavily favour the crammer and the grinder is a disgrace.'

Strong words. Would they seem out of place a century later?

They did not. The demand for a reduction in factual overload continued through the GMC recommendations published in 1957, 1967 and 1980. The GMC deplored the factual overload, the teachers deplored it, the students deplored it – and the factual overload continued to grow. Was this solely the planned obduracy of the medical schools? In part, there was an element of empire building and empire maintenance. But it was more. Advances relevant to medicine have taken place so rapidly and relentlessly over the last 100 years that it was almost inevitable. Who would not want to know about developments such as the structure of enzymes and how they work, the wonders of cell membranes and membrane receptors, the developing field of molecular biology? The biochemists enthused and taught it. Each other traditional specialty similarly enthused and instructed. The psychologists, behavioural scientists, epidemiologists and sociologists also took their new role in a broader-based medicine. Even newer disciplines grew up, teaching the ideas behind informatics and information technology, the ideas behind evidence-based medicine and a dozen other developments. And each discipline added further to the

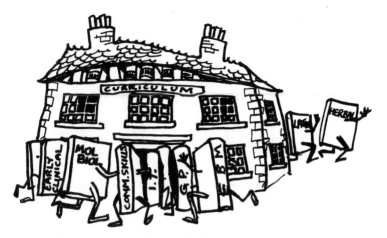

Fig. 3.1 Pressures for curriculum overload are many.

factual information overload, squeezing out the time required for reflection and learning through curiosity. Little was lost from the curriculum while all this accumulated although, true, a knowledge of Latin and of Culpeper's herbal was no longer required (Fig. 3.1). The attitude that 'what is not assessed is not learnt', a self-fulfilling prophecy in the context of such overloaded courses, led to students having 60 or more assessments in the first 2 years of their studies, in an uncoordinated onslaught from multiple course management teams and individuals.

There were related historical reasons for the problem. Centuries ago, medicine was learnt through a clinical apprenticeship. With the growth of understanding of the basic sciences, a preliminary period of scientific training in anatomy, physiology and chemistry/biochemistry was introduced. This formed the preclinical/clinical divide which dominated courses until the recent changes. The second historical reason for overload relates to the Medical Act of 1886, which required that 'the standard of proficiency required from candidates at a qualifying examination shall be such as sufficiently to guarantee the possession of the skill and knowledge required for the practice of medicine, surgery and midwifery'. Qualify today, practice independently tomorrow. Deal with the enteric fever, the crushed limb, the breech delivery. A demanding requirement (Fig. 3.2). A few gained higher qualifications; some gained informal, although often excellent, supervised training, but many did not and there was no requirement to do so. Thus the Medical Act of 1886 had high requirements of the new graduate.

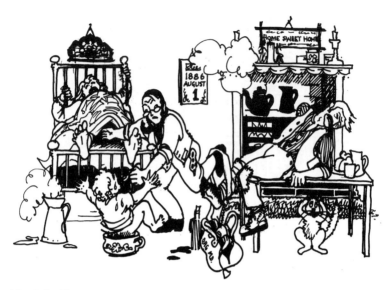

Fig. 3.2 The complete doctor, 1886: 'At least no one can "bleep" me for the next 70 years.'

As a first step towards improving the situation the Goodenough report (1944) recommended the introduction of an extra supervised training year at the end of the then current undergraduate course, and this came to be known as the preregistration year. It was to comprise service under supervision with a significant educational component, and was the responsibility of the university. Its need was reaffirmed in the Todd report (1968), which said that 'The undergraduate medical course does not provide sufficient training for the immediate practice of medicine'. The following Merrison report (1978) noted the failure of the educational component of the preregistration year, and influenced the content of the Medical Act of 1983. Importantly, this now recognized that the aim of producing a new graduate who was competent for independent practice in medicine, surgery and obstetrics was no longer appropriate.

Despite this formal change in the requirements of the new graduate, little changed in the eyes of teachers and examiners. Overload simply grew despite the fact that after registration all doctors need both further training in their chosen specialty and higher qualifications before independent practice is allowed, whether they remain in hospital or choose to become a GP.

Against this background, *Tomorrow's Doctors* set out to change medical education fundamentally. It set out to ensure that all new graduates would have the skills required to adapt to a changing healthcare environment throughout their professional lives, and to update their own learning continually. It set out also to ensure that all graduates would have the necessary knowledge, skills and attitudes required during the preregistration year. And an important feature evident in these most recent recommendations, perhaps lacking previously, is that the GMC would be prepared to use its power under the Medical Act of 1983 to enforce change. It would not only show its teeth but, if necessary, it was prepared to use them.

4

Tomorrow's Doctors: a closer look

Tomorrow's Doctors had 14 principal recommendations. Some of these I would term *developmental* and some I would term *radical*. By 'developmental' I mean recommendations that were closely following current thought in most schools and among many teachers about the need for change. By 'radical' I mean recommendations that would result in a fundamental restructuring of the curriculum, with far-reaching implications. I acknowledge that the overlap between the two categories is considerable, and the division is personal and arbitrary (the possibility of such idiosyncrasy being one of the delights of writing a single-author book). The radical recommendations will be considered at greater length. Not only are they leading to more fundamental change, but they have laid down a pattern for the curriculum which will be outside the experience of the currently qualified doctors with whom you have discussed medical training and a medical career. They therefore have great importance in your understanding of what lies ahead of you. The original numbering of the 14 principal recommendations of *Tomorrow's Doctors*, which are summarized below, is indicated at the end of each proposal in case you want to cross-refer to the original document. This will be available in your medical school library, or may be available from your careers adviser if you are not yet at medical school.

DEVELOPMENTAL PROPOSALS

Summary:

1. Attitudes of mind and behaviour that befit a doctor should be inculcated during training (3).

2. Communication skills should be emphasized throughout the course (8).

3. Theme of public health medicine should figure prominently in the course (9).

4. Teaching should adapt to the changing patterns of health care (10).

5. Learning systems should be informed by modern educational theory and make use of new technology (11).

6. Assessment should match the new-style curriculum (12).

The developmental proposals are considered in detail below.

Attitudes of mind

What attitudes of mind and behaviour befit a doctor? These are discussed in detail in a booklet entitled *Good Medical Practice*, which is essential and expected reading for all medical students. If your medical school does not supply you with a copy, request one – the GMC expects that medical schools will wish to provide a copy for each medical student. The main duties of a doctor are listed in Box 4.1.

Box 4.1   Good medical practice

Make the care of your patient your first concern
Treat every patient politely and considerately
Respect patients' dignity and privacy
Listen to patients and respect their views
Give patients information in a way they can understand
Respect the rights of patients to be fully involved in decisions about their care
Keep your professional knowledge and skills up to date
Recognize the limits of your professional competence
Be honest and trustworthy
Respect and protect confidential information
Make sure that your personal beliefs do not prejudice your patients' care
Act quickly to protect patients from risk if you have good reason to believe that you or a colleague may not be fit to practice
Avoid abusing your position as a doctor
Work with colleagues in ways that best serve patients' interests

---

Communication skills

Deficiencies in this area are responsible for many misunderstandings between patients, relatives, doctors and nursing staff. They occur in the area of written communication as well as that of spoken communication. Medical schools now have courses running through the curriculum as a theme, with the progressive development of communication skills. More on 'themes' in a later section of the book – to me they form the unwritten 15th principal recommendation of *Tomorrow's Doctors*.

Public health

Public health medicine was to have a greater emphasis, with moves towards health promotion and disease prevention as well as the consideration of the role of social factors in disease.

Health care delivery

Health care is increasingly taking place outside the main teaching hospitals, and training should take this into account with more being undertaken in general practice, the community and outlying hospitals. This has major potential resource implications for the traditional teaching hospitals, which receive money known as SIFT money for each clinical medical student. SIFT stands for 'Service Increment For Teaching', and covers all extra costs resulting from hospitals being teaching hospitals. SIFT money, at around £35 000 per clinical student per year in 1997/98, has been the lifebelt that has kept many trust hospitals afloat. The transfer of even a small proportion of SIFT money to teaching elsewhere would cause severe difficulties, and would have to be a gradual process.

Teaching and assessment

There is recognition that the didactic lecture is not usually the best method of learning, that more interactive learning methods should be used, that use should be made of new technology to support developments such as computer-aided learning and that assessment approaches must be appropriate to the new courses being developed. These were all changes already under way, although the use of the lecture for some teaching of large cohorts of students will persist. Not all lectures are dry and didactic.

RADICAL PROPOSALS

7. Factual overload should be substantially reduced (1).
8. Learning should be through curiosity, exploration and critical evaluation (2).
9. Essential required skills are to be acquired under supervision and rigorously assessed (4).
10. Core curriculum should be defined with its essential knowledge, skills and attitudes (5).
11. Special study modules (SSMs) to augment core and allow study in depth (6).
12. Core should be systems-based and integrated (7).

13. New supervisory structures for course management, which should include interdisciplinary membership and junior staff and student representation on committees (13).
14. GMC should ensure implementation of its recommendations...by informal visits...and, when necessary, exercise of its statutory powers (14).

Proposals 7, 10, 11, 12 and 13 are *keystone proposals* (1, 5, 6, 7 and 13). The keystone to *Tomorrow's Doctor* is the reduction of factual overload, and this is to be brought about by the division of the curriculum into two, *core* and *special study modules*. This division is *not* a separation in the sense of the previous preclinical/clinical course. It is a conceptual division, with core and special study modules having different but interrelated functions and frequently running together or with one closely following the other.

Core curriculum

The core will occupy about 65–70% of the curriculum, and will ensure that students have the knowledge, skills and attitudes required of them by the start of the preregistration year. There will be commonality of the core across medical schools, so that a graduate from one medical school will be able to work in a hospital in the normal catchment area of another school. The local employer will know what skills the new doctor will have and new doctors will know that they will not be asked to exercise skills outside their knowledge, training and capability. Schools differ in their traditions and strengths and the opportunities provided by their local populations so that while there will be commonality in the core a 'national' core curriculum will not be sought.

The core will be defined at each medical school, and those deciding what constitutes the core in a given discipline will include scientists and clinicians from both within and outside the discipline, including general practice. Junior doctors and students should be involved in the planning. Preventing the sole decision on content being taken by specialists in the subject, will help to focus the core on essentials and avoid factual overload. Defining the core content is a mammoth task and the GMC says it hasn't the expertise (or the desire) to take it on. Several groups are attempting to define areas of core. There is an effective network and much exchange of information, so that while the core is, in a sense, being defined by individual schools, each is much influenced by other schools.

Core delivery

The planning of teaching and learning objectives by a multi-disciplinary group leads naturally to integrated teaching across disciplines which have traditionally been taught separately. With respect to traditional courses integration is 'vertical', with clinical teaching early in the course and basic science teaching in the later stages. Integration is also 'horizontal'; for instance, renal function would be taught in a coordinated fashion by biochemist, pharmacologist, anatomist and physiologist. The potential advantages for you, as a student, are that it is easier to understand the relevance of the basic sciences when seen in relation to a clinical context, and also easier to understand how the basic sciences themselves are related. Early clinical contact brings additional breadth and interest to the course.

How is this to be brought about? The GMC suggested a 'systems-based' approach to teaching. Examples of 'systems' are the respiratory, cardiovascular and alimentary systems. For instance, if 'asthma' was a topic in part of the course on the respiratory system you would involve: physiologists and anatomists talking about structure, mechanics and gas exchange; biochemists and pharmacologists talking about surfactants, mucus and drug receptors; epidemiologists and toxicologists talking about variations in disease patterns; patients talking about the impact of the disease on their lives, etc. It was apparent to some medical schools that integration would be most appropriately achieved by a case-based or a problem-based approach, rather than by a strictly systems-based approach. For example, if your clinical case concerned someone with cystic fibrosis it was more sensible to consider the effects of the disease on multiple body systems and on the individual, shifting the emphasis from a single system to a whole person. Liverpool and Manchester are medical schools which have designed exciting courses based around clinical cases and problems.

Different approaches to the pattern of delivery of the core throughout the course are possible. Should you start with normality and move on to disease at the population level and its causation before tackling disease in the individual? Should you follow a 'spiral' curriculum, in which, as you progress through the course, the same topic is visited several times at increasing levels of complexity – through normal structure and function to abnormality and clinical practice – first as student and finally at the level of preregistration house officer? A spiral approach was devised and is favoured by Dundee medical school. In truth, it is probably a reduction in factual overload, the definition of the core and good teaching methods that are significant, rather than the exact method or pattern of delivery. Note that simply compressing the current course content into two-thirds of the previously allotted time is not an acceptable way to generate core and free time for SSMs!

Special study modules

While the commonality of core would produce more similar graduates nationwide, the SSMs were intended to produce increased diversity. SSMs are concerned with the long-term intellectual development of the individual rather than the narrower focus of the preregistration year. The implementation of SSMs varies from school to school, and some patterns, guidelines and suggestions will be given in the section on SSMs below. It was intended that SSMs should form part of every year of the course, and although the number and length were not defined it was anticipated that they would occupy about a third of the course, a proportion which many schools are having difficulty in reaching. SSMs are to be assessed as rigorously as the core, despite the difficulty of judging equivalence of standards between very different types of study.

Learning through curiosity

There is to be a change in learning style, which is to become more student-centred, with directed self-learning. This becomes possible with the reduction in factual overload and the development of SSMs. Previously, didactic factual teaching was felt to be the only way to 'get through all that had to be learnt'. These changes are not universally welcomed. Some teachers feel a loss of (perceived) authority. Some students feel a loss of security at not being taught all they need to know. Other students and teachers relish the opportunities and feel it has become easier to learn and teach in an atmosphere of mutual respect.

Acquiring essential skills

My categorization of the acquisition of essential required skills as a radical suggestion may seem strange. However, until recently skills were acquired in an unstructured way and to very variable standards without proper assessment. Thus, some would qualify without knowing how to put up a drip, whereas others would be extremely proficient. Now all those who qualify must have demonstrated a range of skills to a set level of proficiency. A comfort to employing hospitals, patients and the doctors themselves, and one valuable role among many for the clinical skills learning centres (synonym: clinical skills laboratories) now being established in most medical schools.

Implementing the process

The final recommendation: radical because the GMC said that this report *was* to be implemented and that it would take action against medical schools which did not modify their course along the lines indicated. *Tomorrow's Doctors* was not to be a document which medical schools could glance at and set aside with comments such as 'How interesting, but of course we couldn't possibly have that sort of thing here'. This fate had, I suspect, befallen some previous reports.

5

The core curriculum

Just as the GMC shrank back from being the vehicle to define the core, I will make no attempt to define it here – not least because any attempt would both quadruple the length of this book and cause it to go well beyond its purpose.

The core represents the blend of knowledge, skills and attitudes which are considered essential in any medical graduate. Courses used to be overloaded as a result of the enthusiasm of the lecturers for their subject, but their core content is now to be defined by what is required of the newly graduated student. This means that from the start of each section of the course you will know what you will be expected to have gained by the end. You can expect better documentation to help you meet the aims and objectives of the course, more structured teaching, and also more responsibility for covering specified areas not formally covered by your tutor or in clinical work. Defining the core puts a boundary round the learning that you need. It is not intended to stifle your enthusiasm for exploring areas you happen to find of particular interest, and a well defined core will leave room for such exploration.

To illustrate the sort of information that a student can expect, I will use examples from the Paediatric module offered at Leeds. This was devised by Dr Murdoch-Eaton, Consultant Senior Lecturer in Paediatrics and Medical Education. The course is described in a 16-page booklet given to each student at the start of the attachment. The course starts with an introductory week, providing teaching on key topics: normal growth and development, the paediatric history, an introduction to disability as it affects children and their families and, as stated, 'the delights of examining babies and children'. The aims, objectives, teaching methods and timetable of each part of the course are given. Teaching locations include hospital wards and clinics in the main teaching hospital, a DGH (District General Hospital) attachment and work in the community. As well as giving learning objectives, the booklet specifies what are *not* learning objectives. For example, a visit to a special needs school takes place. Its purpose is for the students to mix with and learn to communicate with children with special needs, and to understand the pressures and demands on their families – not to learn all the physical signs and biochemical abnormalities associated with numerous rare syndromes. The aims of the course, in terms of knowledge and skills, are clearly given.

Examples of knowledge aims are:

- to develop an understanding of why paediatrics is not the same as 'medicine in small adults'
- to develop an understanding of the normal changes during the growth and development of children
- to acquire a basic knowledge of common childhood illnesses and problems
- to develop an understanding of local services available for children.

Examples of skills aims are:

- to develop an ability to relate to children
- to develop skills of examining babies and children
- to make a reasonable differential diagnosis of illnesses and problems in babies and children
- to develop communication and counselling skills.

Each teaching location provides different, though often overlapping, learning oppotunities, and these are made clear in the objectives listed for each part of the course. For example, the students know that during the community week they will have sessions with a health visitor, a visit to a well-baby clinic and work with a child development assessment team. The students also know that one of the listed objectives will require self-directed learning on normal child development and its variations, followed by practice under supervision by personal tutors.

The booklet also tells students the content of the core curriculum, in terms of the topics about which they will be expected to have knowledge and may be examined. This makes it clear to students that they will not see all the required conditions during their clinical work, nor will all the topics be covered in formal teaching and tutorials. Much of the core is defined in terms of problems that the student will be expected to be able to discuss. The level of knowledge required is similar to that in other areas which have been formally taught. The types of problem are varied, but cover the important and common areas of paediatric care. Examples of case problems might require students to outline the diagnosis, investigation and management of:

- a 2-month-old baby presenting with a 48-hour history of vomiting
- a boy aged 12 months with an undescended testis
- an unwell, pyrexial 5-year-old with a purpuric rash (management from point of view of GP, admitting doctor and community physician)
- a 6-year-old who has recently developed a limp.

As well as defining the core and what is expected of the student, the booklet provides information on the methods of assessment used during and at the end of the course, the personal tutor support system and how the student may provide feedback on the course. The paediatric core curriculum is followed, and must be passed, by all students, but they also have the opportunity to study paediatrics further during an SSM.

The above is one example of part of a core curriculum. Each section of your course should have a defined core, with fairly detailed learning objectives, as well as there being overall aims and objectives related to the core content of the whole course. Having a properly defined core helps to limit factual overload and to focus teaching, learning and assessment. The core is complemented by SSMs, and both are exciting and important in their own right. It is to SSMs that we move next.

6

Special study modules (SSMs)

Tomorrow's Doctors has two major paragraphs outlining the scope and purpose of SSMs:

- Para 24: '...the greatest educational opportunities will be affordable by the part of the course which goes beyond the limits of the core, that allows students to study in depth in areas of particular interest to them, that provides them with insights into scientific method and the discipline of research and that engenders an approach to medicine that is constantly questioning and self-critical...'
- Para 31: '...we would expect approximately one third of the total undergraduate programme to be devoted to them. We would hope that at all stages of the course students will be engaged in some work outside the core syllabus but schools may wish to set aside blocks of time for special studies. They may also choose to require students to undertake at least one study from each of a number of subject groupings...'.

SSMs were a new idea and are still being explored, developed and changed. They pose quite an organizational challenge, as a simple calculation shows. Many SSMs are suitable for only a small number of students, perhaps one to four, to take at the same time – so for each student to take one SSM you might need 100 or more projects a year for a cohort of 200 students. For two SSMs per year throughout the 5 years of a typical course, this is the equivalent of 1000 project places each year by the time SSMs have worked their way up through all the years of the course! The pattern, timing and number of SSMs offered varies between schools, but the following will give you an idea of the scope available and some of the things to think about in choosing your SSMs. On a typical 5-year course study time is about 180–190 weeks; allowing one-third for SSMs gives them about 60 weeks. After deducting a 12-week elective, we are left with 48 weeks, or approximately 10 weeks/year, or the equivalent, devoted to SSMs. Two common patterns of SSM are the *long, thin* and the *short, fat*. By 'long, thin' I mean the study period runs alongside other studies for a term or a year at, say, half a day/week. By 'short, fat' I mean essentially your whole time is devoted to the project. 'Short' is relative – it could be a few days, or a couple of months. Sometimes a long, thin SSM could be scheduled as a short, fat SSM, or vice versa, but not always.

Let's look at a couple of examples. An example of a long, thin SSM would involve following a pregnancy from confirmation of conception, through delivery to the 3-month stage postpartum. Spread to half a day twice/month over a year, this time could be used as a basis for looking at lots of issue (see Box 6.1).

Box 6.1 Long, thin SSM in 'Pregnancy, childbirth and the first three months'

Fetal development
Health issues (smoking, alcohol, diet, breastfeeding)
Social issues (income changes, costs)
Family issues (effects on other children, husband–wife relationship, extended
    family support)
Body image issues (changes in pregnancy and puerperium)
Child development in first 3 months
Contraception
Any other issues you wish to explore

A second example is an SSM requiring you to write a 3000-word review, given one afternoon of dedicated time per week over 10 weeks. Topics could be very varied, e.g. 'A critical evaluation of recent changes in medical education', 'The role of the physician in literature', 'Modern management of diabetic eye disease'. You would learn skills such as using libraries and searching electronic databases, how to write literature references, how to structure arguments in an essay, how to write to length and how to keep to schedule. Note that these three essay-based projects all develop the same sorts of skill despite their very different nature. One advantage is that you are tackling a topic which you have chosen because it interests you. This is an example in which the focus is on the *process* of what you are doing rather than the *content*, although the latter may be fascinating as well.

Examples of short, fat modules are working in a laboratory learning about tissue culture methods or molecular biology techniques. Clinical projects, such as working in a discipline not routinely covered in your school's clinical studies, are included, for example plastic and reconstructive surgery. In these examples both the content and the process vary, but the overall function of the SSM – to add breadth and insight – is achieved.

One of the principles underlying SSMs is choice. This is not absolute, and will be regulated. It may be regulated by availability. For example, if 20 students opt for a medical journalism option with a capacity of two, 90% will be disappointed. (So enquire early and keep your own counsel.) Choice may be regulated by a requirement to undertake SSMs in a particular order or of a particular type. For example, early on all students may have to do a literature search/write-up type of SSM to ensure that they have the basic library skills required for later parts of the course. On the other hand, you may not be allowed to take an SSM on bereavement counselling during the first year because it is considered you have insufficient clinical experience to benefit from it. The school may impose other restrictions to ensure that your SSMs collectively exhibit breadth, as suggested in paragraph 31 of *Tomorrow's Doctors*, quoted above. Schools may define subject areas in each year of the course which have to be tackled through an SSM. A hypothetical example is shown in Box 6.2.

Box 6.2   SSMs through the course (hypothetical example)

Year	SSM 1	SSM 2	SSM 3
1	Literature/essay	Clinical topic	HIV-related project
2	Public health/IT	Free choice	Project with external body
3	Free choice	Health screening	Wider-context project
4	Basic science	Ethical issues	Basic science/clinical project
5	Community project	Elective period	Free choice (extended elective)

Your school may also link the SSMs with the specialties you are studying in a given year. For example, if the SSM is to be on an ethics-related issue in Year 4, and you have attachments in general practice and paediatrics in that year, you may be expected to develop your ethics SSM in one of those areas, not least because it will be easier to arrange supervision and support.

Think hard about how you can make best use of your SSMs and what you want to get out of them. Do you want to sample many unrelated areas to give maximum breadth? Do you want to avoid laboratory-based basic science SSMs? Do you want to take SSMs in areas that you definitely do *not* want to pursue as a future career? For example, if you are already a committed clinical microbiologist, a period in primary care would provide insight into what their diagnostic problems were in microbiology. If you do not want breadth, do you want to build a portfolio of related SSMs which could help you with postregistration job applications? If keen on respiratory disease, your essay-related SSM could be on asthma, as could your clinical topic in Year 1. Your Year 2 public health SSM could look at epidemiological factors and pollutants, your Year 4 basic science SSM could look at smooth muscle receptors and bronchoconstriction, and so on. Even if your career intentions change as you go through the medical course, you will have built up expertise in an area and had the thrill of making often unexpected insights, which is so rewarding.

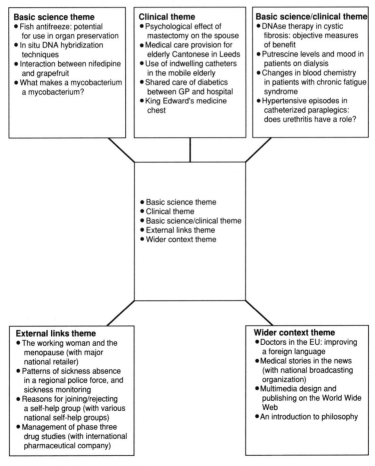

Fig. 6.1 Sample types of SSM.

SSMs are many and varied. Look at Fig. 6.1 to appreciate the flavour of this variety. Remember that many schools allow you to devise and arrange your own SSMs to reflect your own interests, as long as the learning objectives set out in *Tomorrow's Doctors* for SSMs are met.

7

Intercalated degrees and electives

These two traditional parts of the medical course will be retained in the new curriculum of most medical schools.

INTERCALATED DEGREES

Most schools encourage some of their students to study a subject related to their course as a pure discipline for an academic year. Generally this has been in a science-based subject, such as biochemistry, histology or psychology, leading to an honours degree in the chosen discipline. Some students in the future may look more widely to subjects such as ethics or information technology, or even business and management studies or a modern European language. The advantages of intercalating a degree are that you have an opportunity to study a subject in depth which you find interesting. It will help prepare those wishing to pursue an academic/ research career and in your early post-qualification years may strengthen a job application to an academic unit. The disadvantages can be considerable. Almost certainly, you will not be given a grant and will have to pay your course fees. While reduced or zero fees were often charged for intercalating students in the past, in the current financial climate universities are tending to charge fees at the full rate. These are obviously severe financial disincentives. You will be a student for an extra year. This is either an advantage or a disadvantage depending on your point of view, but a few years down the track the extra time will seem irrelevant whatever your immediate perspective. If you wish to intercalate enquire early, at least 1 year ahead, as some schools have bursaries to support intercalating students and these are limited in number. If possible, ensure that you are performing academically in the top third of the cohort and that you do not need to resit any subjects. Imperial College, London, which has an immensely strong science tradition, proposes a variant of the intercalated degree. All its students will take a modular BSc degree course, spread through a 6-year undergraduate course. This may avoid some of the funding difficulties associated with the intercalated degree.

ELECTIVES

The elective is a traditional and much enjoyed part of most medical courses. Electives generally take place in the later part of the course. They vary in length from a few weeks to a few months, and will fall in the section of the course devoted to SSMs. While some students stay in their home institution, most use the opportunity to study abroad or elsewhere in the UK. When choosing an elective, first check what your institution offers and what help is given in making the arrangements. Before arranging a do-it-yourself elective with a great-aunt's cousin twice removed who lives in Borneo, check the requirements of your medical school regarding a valid elective. Do you need a defined project? What sort of report is required? Do you have to be based in an academic institution? If you have an elective period of 3 months can you work half the time in an institution and spend half the time touring round the country?

Allow plenty of time to make all the arrangements. The administrative officer or academic involved in arranging electives should be able to advise, but expect it to take 6 months for all but the most straightforward elective. Finally, look at your exam and firm schedules and keep up with your work. It is sad to see students sitting at home having to repeat a course or resit an exam when they should be enjoying themselves on an elective. Receiving postcards from friends in exotic places saying 'Wish you were here' just isn't the same.

8

Themes

There are 14 principal recommendations listed in *Tomorrow's Doctors*. If there had been 15, the extra one would have related to themes within the curriculum. Within the systems-based course proposed, the GMC considered that there were a number of defined themes which should permeate the system-based and topic-based courses that constitute the core (see Box 8.1).

Box 8.1   GMC themes

Clinical method
Communication skills
Human biology
Human disease
Man in society
The public health
Handicap, disability and rehabilitation
Research and experiment

Different medical schools have adopted different approaches to themes to suit their own individual character, but generally encompass the GMC's themes in one form or another. Note particularly the inclusion of human biology and of research and experiment. From the earliest deliberations on *Tomorrow's Doctors*, the GMC set out to allay the fear of many basic scientists and clinicians that there was to be a watering down of the scientific content of the new curriculum, and an associated move from 'education' to 'training'. The GMC explicitly states that 'It is appropriate to emphasize... that the curriculum changes that we recommend are intended to strengthen the scientific component of the course and certainly not to weaken it'. No reduction in *relevant and appropriate* basic science is intended. As with other aspects of the curriculum, the difficulty is often in judging what is 'relevant and appropriate' at undergraduate level, and in deciding who should make that judgement.

'Man in society' refers to courses already present in many medical schools, covering things such as human development, ethics, sociology and psychology relevant to medicine. While the topics are all valuable as themes, the traditional title for such courses is not a happy one in a predominantly female world! Gender-neutral alternatives are being adopted.

As mentioned, Dundee's course has a spiral curriculum, with core and special study modules. Running through the course and contributing to their systems-based programme are 21 themes (see Box 8.2). As well as running through the programme, some themes have a course built around them for further in-depth study. You can see clearly how the Dundee themes cross-link with those suggested by the GMC.

Box 8.2 The 21 Dundee themes		
Acute care	Anatomy	Behaviour
Biochemistry	Child health	Clinical method (includes communication)
The community	Computers and IT	Disability and rehabilitation
Genetics	Health promotion/ public health	Infectious disease
Investigative procedures	Medical ethics	Microbiology
Oncology	Pathology	Physiology
Research method/statistics	Surgery	Therapeutics/ pharmacology

The identification of themes benefits both student and teacher. For example, explicitly identifying ethical issues makes it easier to compare different approaches in different specialties to issues which, when viewed together, are seen to have much in common. Ethical issues related to patient autonomy arise in many specialties, and linkage within a theme emphasizes how they are interrelated (see Box 8.3).

One common factor you will note is that there is often not a clear-cut answer which balances the rights of the individual, including that to medical confidentiality, with those of others and of society as a whole. Think about some of these issues, choosing ones which require little medical background, and see if your conclusions and those of a colleague are similar. If not, why not?

Do they reflect differences in gender, religious belief, culture or ethnicity? Would you be prepared to compromise? Does the concept of a 'correct' view hold?

Themes also help course planners to avoid both the omission of important issues and the duplication of less important ones. Some schools, such as Leeds, have individuals responsible for the major themes who work with the various multidisciplinary course management teams to ensure that specific themes are adequately represented and are covered coherently over the programme of study.

Box 8.3   Issues of patient autonomy

Request for 'social' abortion of one of two twins
Sterilization without consent of spouse
Continued smoking by a young family man with heart disease
Discharge against medical advice
Refusal of 'appropriate' informed consent
Request for euthanasia
Refusal to disclose positive HIV status to partner
Driving when known to be under influence of drugs/alcohol
Request by spouse not to tell partner diagnosis of cancer

9

Planning and learning

Before looking at how we can learn best in the different situations met on the medical course, I want to look briefly at two quite general areas – planning study time and thinking about the actual process of learning. We also need to look at a little educational terminology which often leads to confusion, and at what is meant by problem-based learning (PBL) and case-based learning.

The methods you use to plan your time and the way you study may differ from those discussed below. If your methods work for you and you feel they will meet the demands of the course, then stick to them. If you have concerns then consider what follows. Remember, though, that what worked at A level or the equivalent may not be able to cope with the demands of a university course.

PLANNING STUDY AND LEISURE TIME

How do you plan your study time? Is it by the week, month, semester, term or year? Most students plan by a combination of these, using the week as the basic unit but being aware of events and deadlines that appear on a longer timescale for exams, essays, project work, etc. Box 9.1 is a weekly chart which can be copied and used as a timetable. If you want a larger copy, use a photocopier that allows enlargements. Enter in your fixed commitments such as lectures, practicals and tutorials and then decide when you are going to fit in private study. Try to study at times when you know you are most receptive to learning. The timetable covers the early morning and the late night, recognizing that people's study habits vary – you are not expected to be studying from early morning until late at night. While the number of hours students study varies, during an average week the total of fixed commitments and concentrated private study should probably not exceed 40–45 hours. If you are finding that you regularly need more than 50 hours to keep up, then discusss things with friends and a tutor as you may need some guidance about either technique or what is actually required of you. If you include planned leisure time on the timetable, it will help you to get the balance right and give you some highlights during the week to look forward to.

Box 9.1   Timetable for study and leisure

WEEKLY PLAN: STARTING DATE   /   /

	Mon	Tues	Wed	Thu	Fri	Sat	Sun
6–8 h							
8–9 h							
9–10 h							
10–11 h							
11–12 h							
12–13 h							
13–14 h							
14–15 h							
15–16 h							
16–17 h							
17–18 h							
18–19 h							
19–20 h							
20–21 h							
21–22 h							
22–23 h							
23–24 h							
24–01 h							

Timetables are for guidance only. Use them sensibly. Some weeks you may do extra and at other times you may miss a couple of sessions. After a few weeks compare how much time work is taking compared with planned time and adjust accordingly. Essays, for example, commonly take more time than planned. As well as planning your weekly schedule, think about a wall-chart for the whole year so that you don't get caught out by deadlines for work or by the exams arriving with unexpected abruptness.

INDIVIDUAL STUDY

If you ask members of staff how students learn they come up with statements like '...mainly from lectures and tutorials, but also from practical sessions...'. If you ask a student the perspective is often rather different: '...mostly on my own in the library or my flat, although some of the tutorials are good'. This section is about individual study, how to go about it and what its problems are. Certainly for all of you, study outside the confines of the lecture theatre and tutorial room will form a major part of your learning. Some of the first things to sort out are the '*where*', '*when*' and '*for how long*' of individual study.

The '*where*' is perhaps the easiest of the three, and is a 'condition' rather than a 'place'. It should be where you feel comfortable studying, where you can concentrate and where you can have your books and other study materials around you. For most this will be in your study-bedroom or flat or in the library. Enjoy the coffee bar or students' common room, but don't fool yourself that either is the place for serious study. If you use your own room, set it up to your own liking with adequate light and heating and books, files etc. close at hand. Many find it helps their concentration to have one area specifically associated with study.

The '*when*' is easier for you to define than for me. Different people study best at different times of day. Some work best in the early evening or early morning, others late at night. Having studied for university entrance you will know what suited you best: guard that time carefully, because prime time is a most precious commodity. Make sure that you use some of it most days for concentrated periods of study. Whatever time of day or night you work best, make sure that you get enough sleep. As noted above, be sensible. Regularly working from 6–8 o'clock in the morning is fine, but not if you stay up beyond midnight every night.

'*For how long?*' Learning is an active process, and despite the tales that you will hear few people are able to *concentrate* for more than an hour at a time without a break, and most for considerably less. Plan short breaks. Five to ten minutes' complete break will renew your concentration and allow you to absorb and understand more material. Make it a complete break. Have a coffee, talk to the budgerigar or get a breath of fresh air. Plan how long you are going to spend overall studying in a session and try to stick roughly to it. Use a timetable as outlined above to help plan your time.

Time or topic

Should you study just 'time' or 'topic?' I would strongly suggest the latter. Don't aim for '2 hours work' but aim 'to understand and be able to draw the Krebs' cycle'. This approach allows you to set and achieve realistic goals. The alternative approach can lead to staring at a page for minutes at a time with nothing going in.

The 'studying topic' approach should be made an active approach. Write down what you know to start with, list the main points of what you want to know and then sketch in the more detailed bits. Divide the knowledge into levels: 'must know', 'should know' and 'nice to know'. '*Must know*' knowledge is the framework of knowledge required to understand the topic and proceed further. '*Should know*' knowledge adds breadth and is often helpful in tying topics together. '*Nice to know*' knowledge may be an anecdote or a piece of medical history (e.g. 'Who was Krebs?') that you can well survive without. When you are close to the end of your session, review what you have covered for a few minutes and tie it in with anything else you are learning. We may tend to teach physiology, anatomy and biochemistry separately but they are more easily understood when considered together.

The bad times

All sounds easy, doesn't it? But then there are the bad times when you don't feel like work, nothing is going in and you ask what is the relevance of it all anyway. It all becomes too much. Realistically, these times occur. While there are no magic solutions, here are some suggestions which others have found helpful.

The first step in studying is often the most difficult. If you are having difficulty starting, then choose something constructive but straightforward, e.g. write down the main points of the last lecture or tutorial. If you are having difficulty with a topic, look at another book. It may contain a better diagram or explanation. If you are finding that mini-breaks are not restoring your concentration, ask yourself if you are bored with what you are studying. Mini-breaks help concentration but they rarely overcome boredom. Two approaches to boredom: alternate the topic that bores you, in short sections, with ones which interest you; or find a friend and get him/her to teach you the topic in the style of your favourite lecturer. Explaining topics to each other is a good way for both to learn.

None of this may work. Remember your overall aim is to qualify as a good doctor, and try to stick with it. Discuss things with one of your tutors if you seem to be having a lot more difficulty than your fellow students. This will be seen as a sign of common sense not weakness. They are there to help. Finally, some find that mild shock treatment is a great stimulus. Try answering questions off a previous exam paper under near exam conditions.

DEEP AND SURFACE LEARNING

Pick up any general textbook on psychology and you will find many complex theories of learning. Those of you who have studied psychology at A level will be aware of many of these, and their substantiation using rats running through mazes and pigeons feeding on corn. These theories are often difficult to relate to the everyday experience of being a student. Among them you may find a small gem, a discussion of *deep* and *surface* learning.

Surface learning is an approach to learning characterized by the memorization of the detail of, and information in, a book or lecture. *Deep* learning is characterized by its focus being on the overall structure of the information and the way it fits into and extends an existing framework of knowledge and understanding. It looks at the big picture and fits it into the even bigger picture.

Asked about studying, surface learners make comments like:

— 'I get down most of the lists they give you in lectures and remember those'
— 'Cramming seems best for me, I only remember the things I've learnt the day before the exam, the rest is just beer time'
— 'I collect dozens of facts and keep on writing them down and then in the exams try to make them fit into the questions'.

Deep learners say things like:

— 'I write down the main principles and try to fit them into what else I know'
— 'I try to fit it into a practical example – it can be difficult but you suddenly get these flashes of understanding and it all drops into place. Then it's not a matter of learning it, it just becomes part of what you know'.

Until arriving at university, it will have been possible to study and succeed in exams using either approach. *From now on, a surface approach becomes increasingly inappropriate.* The volume and complexity of new material means that a deep approach is required for success. Indeed, to integrate theory with clinical signs and symptoms, in order to make a correct diagnosis, itself requires that you adopt a deep approach to learning.

Pause for a moment and consider the approach that you adopted when you last revised for exams. Surface, deep or combined? A surface approach is not always inappropriate. We all use a surface approach at times for remembering lists. Examples are mnemonics for the colours in the rainbow or, in a medical context, the (risqué) mnemonics used by countless generations of students to remember the sequence of the 12 cranial nerves. What is important is that we adopt the deep approach to most of our learning. This is why time and again throughout this guide there is an emphasis on the overall structure of a topic and the way it relates to material already learnt. Independent research has demonstrated the value of the deep approach. Elsewhere in this guide, in the section on 'Good Writing', is a discussion of the SOLO taxonomy. This is a system, which can be applied across a wide range of degree courses, used to judge the quality of written work. Students whose written work was good enough to earn a first or upper second class honours degree all used a deep approach to learning. Third class honours graduates had used a surface approach. Enough said? Of course, the good news is that you can learn to adopt a deep approach to your studies even if up to now you have succeeded largely by using a surface approach. That is largely what much of this guide is about: the quality of learning and how it should be promoted.

Unfortunately, the nature of much of medical school education has until now been such that surface learning has been encouraged. Factors which encourage a surface learning approach include courses concentrating on facts without overall concepts, volume overload and multiple assessments, such that everything ends up being learnt 'because it will be examined' and nothing is learnt for its intrinsic value. One of the reasons for the move to the core curriculum plus special study modules is to try to combat this built-in pressure on students to adopt a surface learning approach by both reducing volume overload and giving students time to focus on areas which they find particularly interesting. It's encouraging, but there are pressures in the other direction from those who believe that 'only what is assessed is learnt'. Unfortunately, powerful Course Review Committees sometimes fall into this group.

The 'only what is assessed is learnt' view of students and education is depressing to me. Most of you will be accomplished to some extent at sport, music or some other hobby. You are unlikely to have worked to learn this skill because 'you were to be assessed' but persevered because of your intrinsic interest in it. Fortunately, the high standard of work that I see produced in special study modules supports the view that intrinsic interest can be the driving force to quality work and learning, and that the role of assessment is secondary. This gives me great cheer.

CASE-BASED AND PROBLEM-BASED LEARNING (PBL)

Let's move on to the final topic in this chapter – educational terminology – and the often confused terms case-based learning and problem-based learning. Also, we will look at why it is important that you are aware of the confusion and know the difference between the two terms, which are frequently, although wrongly, used interchangeably. As we will see they are different, although both refer to valuable learning methods.

The principles of case-based learning will be familiar to you through the study of subjects such as physics at school. You are taught principles of physics, such as Newton's laws of motion, and then you apply these to certain problems in order to check and aid your understanding. The problems ensure that you can apply the theoretical knowledge that you have learnt and that you truly understand it. The reinforcement that takes place, and the change from abstract concept to concrete examples, helps the learning. The order is theoretical knowledge first, application to examples second. In the context of a medical course, in case-based learning you have extensive pre-existing knowledge in the area and apply it to the clinical case scenario. Using the established knowledge base plus additional resources you learn from the case. This usually involves finding the diagnosis, considering the differential diagnosis or arranging a management strategy. Again, the reinforcement of theoretical knowledge and its application to a real clinical case help learning. Overall, it is an effective and enjoyable way of learning and is one way of bringing early clinical contact into the curriculum. Because the clinical cases are usually seen as 'problems' and their purpose is often to encourage 'solving of the problem', for instance making a diagnosis, they are often called 'problem-based learning'. As noted above, this is wrong – true problem-based learning is an educational approach with many important differences. So, if you visit a school which says its course has a 'problem-based learning' approach, make sure you know whether they are talking about 'case-based learning' or true 'problem-based learning', as discussed below. Students who are happy with the one approach may be unhappy with the other.

Problem-based learning (PBL) is a system of medical education pioneered and developed in centres including McMaster University, Canada, and the University of Newcastle, New South Wales. The learning sequence is very different from that in traditional medical courses and courses with a case-based component. Before looking at the process of PBL take 5 minutes to think about the following PBL problem. The sample problem is simple. You are given a photo of two adults who are grossly obese. You are told that they are twin sisters in their thirties. Draw a mind-map of all the learning issues you could tackle starting from this problem. (If you are not used to mind-maps, take a blank sheet of A4 paper sideways on. Draw a box in the middle containing the words 'obese twin sisters' and from that draw lines radiating out to boxes indicating any relevent issues you can think of. Some of these issues may have sub-issues – similarly, draw lines out from main issue boxes to sub-issue boxes. This makes up the start of a mind-map.)

The essentials of the process of PBL are:

1. *The problem is the first stage in the learning sequence.* There is no prior induction or preparation.

2. The presentation of the problem is as it would be in real life.

3. The student (or, more commonly, group of students) identifies appropriate learning issues to explore and decides which need to be tested and evaluated.

4. An initial cycle of study results in the solution of some issues and the identification of further issues, which are brought back to the group and discussed.

5. The cycle is repeated as often as is fruitful. Individual students may tackle all issues or some issues may be tackled by just some members of the group and reported to the others. Some issues may represent individual, rather than group, learning goals.

6. The learning that has taken place while studying the problem is integrated into the knowledge base of each individual student.

Note the major differences here. The *student* identifies the issues and learning objectives. It is self-directed learning. Learning is also an open process and different students tackling the same problem will set different learning objectives, partly because they may be at different stages of the course but mainly because they have different needs.

How did you manage with the sample problem? You may have a fairly well filled sheet of paper. A few issues in my mind-map were: genetic predisposition, physiological control of appetite (sub-issue: appetite-suppressant drugs), cultural and social factors, body image ideas (sub-issue: anorexia nervosa), role of diabetes in obesity and vice versa, osteoarthritis, physiology of fat metabolism (sub-issue: something about brown fat and weight control), life insurance. You could explore all these issues and many more, greatly expanding your knowledge base, but the 'problem' of the cause or management of the twins' obesity is not solved. This does not matter from the point of view of the learning exercise.

Note that the student does not need a pre-existing knowledge base in this area. In fact it is seen as a disadvantage as it confines ideas. Formal lectures may not be used at all in a PBL course, although some courses use them for things such as updates in rapidly developing areas, or when they have an expert visitor who is used to presenting material in that way. (Antipathy to lectures may be so strong that in some schools they avoid the term 'lecture' – they become 'occasional large group educational exchange sessions' or something similar!)

PBL is student-centred and self-directed. Once the student has become experienced at it, there is no need for tutor input in identifying learning objectives. Early on there will be some guidance to ensure certain important issues are identified and to ensure that the students do not stray too far outside the bounds of the curriculum. Hours spent on the detailed physics of cardiac ultrasound would not be good use of time in the problem of a heart murmur found in a woman in an antenatal clinic.

A number of educational advantages are claimed for PBL (see Box 9.2)

Box 9.2   Educational advantages of PBL

Clinical reasoning skills developed
Information from many disciplines integrated
Students see their learning as relevant
Students develop lifelong learning skills
Overlap between problems leads to reinforcement
Learning is student-centred and self-directed
Students are treated as adult developing professionals and they respond
  appropriately

Critics of PBL say that you cannot prove that you get a better doctor at the end of it all, major gaps can be left in students' knowledge and their basic science training is less good. In practice graduates from PBL schools such as McMaster and Newcastle, NSW, are highly sought after in a competitive employment market. Supporters of PBL point out that even if graduates of PBL courses were only as good as the products of conventional courses, students seem to enjoy the PBL type of course a lot more and that makes them worthwhile.

Many new medical schools around the world are being set up on PBL lines. New medical schools have been proposed for the UK and it is likely that these will have an emphasis on a PBL curriculum, as well as more community-based teaching. Established medical schools are undergoing further cycles of curriculum reform, and some may go down the PBL route rather than just the case-based learning route. A major concern has been that PBL is demanding of staff time because work is in small groups rather than in large lectures theatres, but institutions offering established PBL courses do not take this view.

A truly PBL course will give you a very different kind of experience from one which calls itself a PBL course but really has a case-based and problem-solving approach. One is not intrinsically better than the other but some students will prefer a certain approach and all students will not be suited by either. So, if told a school has a PBL course a little discreet clarification is required before you either rule it out or rule it in as a place to apply to.

10 Learning from lectures

The 50–60-minute lecture still dominates many courses which deal with large numbers of students. Lectures have the reputation of being soporific events concerned solely with the transmission of facts better obtained from a textbook. Not true. You will learn much from lectures if you tackle them in a constructive manner and the designers of your course understand both their potential and their problems.

Uses of the lecture include:

- providing an overview/summary of an area
- highlighting and discussing difficult areas
- covering and linking areas not well covered in standard text books
- talking about relevant research topics and recent discoveries.

How do you get the most out of lectures? First, by understanding and acknowledging their limitations, which are several and various. They frequently take place in semi-darkness in a stuffy, airless lecture theatre. This and their length can indeed make them soporific. Although experienced, very few lecturers are formally trained as teachers so material may be less well structured than that you are used to. The number of students involved often inhibits and limits opportunities for discussion, making communication seem purely one-way. A few lecturers will use techniques to overcome these limitations but many will not. Second, you need to be well prepared and understand that 'listening' is an active process.

Preparation

1. Know the lecture topic in advance.
2. Spend a few minutes before the lecture mapping out areas that you would expect the lecture to cover. You will be surprised what you already know.

3. Don't arrive late. You may miss the lecture outline or links to previous lectures. You may miss being told what won't be covered. Being late is in any case impolite to both your colleagues and the lecturer.

4. Sit near the front, where you can see and hear easily, and sit with a group with whom you feel at ease. If the lecturer uses small group discussions to break up the lecture, these are then more productive (and fun).

Active listening

Many lecturers use a standard format for their lecture. Awareness of this helps understanding and note-taking. In essence it is 'Tell 'em what you're going to tell, tell it, then tell 'em what you told 'em'. More formally, outline of lecture, body of lecture and summary. Look for these areas, transitions between them and any links with other areas.

Taking notes

Note-taking in lectures is a personal matter but there are some basic considerations, outlined below:

1. Be selective. Any attempt at writing down everything said will both fail and prevent you from understanding the lecture.

2. Take legible notes. There is not time to copy out all your notes after each lecture to make them legible.

3. Reinforce. Studies suggest that you will remember under half the lecture content when you leave the lecture theatre. After 1 week you will remember only half of this. Ten minutes spent the evening after a lecture can prevent much of this loss and save you a great deal of work later. Read through your notes, put them aside, sketch out a summary of main areas, subheadings and examples from the lecture. Check back. Amend. Repeat once. Mark anything you don't understand and check in your textbook or ask a fellow student. Use half a page at the end of each lecture for providing links with other lectures or information. It is these links which make the various subjects – anatomy, physiology, clinical medicine – understandable, rather than just lists of dissociated information, ideas and facts, if you are not on a properly integrated course.

Note-taking itself needs practice. It is easier if you realize that a lecture contains a variety of components of varying relevance. These are glorified by the bizarre acronym 'POKE EARS' (see Box 10.1).

Box 10.1   POKE EARS

P – Preamble
O – Orientation
K – Key points
E – Extensions

E – Examples
A – Asides
R – Reservations
S – Summaries

Preamble is simply brief introductory comment. The *Orientation* tells you what will be covered and how, and ties this lecture in with other parts of the course. *Key points* are the major areas around which the lecture is structured and these should be recorded along with the *Extensions*, which are the secondary areas covered and often related to that Key point. *Examples* provide useful illustrations of a given point to help understanding and should be distinguished from *Asides*, which have less relevance but may be used to introduce light relief or humour or to provide transition between topics. *Reservations* are limitations on the validity of a given argument and *Summaries* are used to bring together a subsection of a lecture or a whole topic. Listen for key phrases which mark the above. Examples are 'There are three areas to cover today…' (Orientation); 'Let us look at a typical case…' (Example); 'The major thing to understand is that…' (Key point); '…but in very severe asthma the child may no longer wheeze' (Reservation); 'Hello, I am Dr Jekyll' (Preamble). POKE EARS, and its value to lecturer and lecturee, was originally described by George Brown, an educationalist from Nottingham.

Notes should follow the structure of the lecture. Indent notes so that information stays together. Thus:

Lecture is covering Key point A, Key point B, Key point C.

> Key point A. Description.
>> Extension 1 to Key point A. Description.
>> First Example to Extension 1.
>> Second Example to Extension 1.

> Key point B. Description.

Etc.

Underline, use CAPITALS or **asterisks** to highlight features.

Some students find it useful to use only one side of a page for lecture notes, using the facing page for any additional notes, diagrams or links and references made later. While the above applies specifically to lectures, a similar structure to notes made from textbooks is equally valuable.

Do not under any circumstances attempt to keep lecture notes on individual loose sheets. They must be kept in a ring-binder or the equivalent. Otherwise at the end of the first term you will have one thousand sheets of chaos. I have known students fail courses because they have been unable to organize themselves to organize notes.

Exchange notes with a friend a few times and compare what you have selected. Ask yourself if you missed out things important to you, and if so why. Remember that the lecture is not over when you leave the lecture theatre. The reinforcement discussed above is most important and over your years as a student will save you much valuable time.

Most lecturers provide an opportunity for questions either during the lecture or on an individual basis after the lecture. Don't be afraid to ask – they are there to help. If you are having difficulties with a given lecturer, then discuss these with him/her constructively. He/she may not realize that the overhead projections are not legible from beyond the front row, or that you cannot take notes from the slides as the lecture theatre is blacked out. Be positive in your suggestions.

Finally, remember lecturers are human too: a smile or friendly word can help a lecturer relax and give a better lecture, to everyone's benefit. Talking to a sea of blank faces giving no feedback can be pretty daunting to most of us!

Enjoy lectures and use the advice above to make the most of them.

11
Effective reading

Textbooks have an almost organic tendency to multiply and grow from edition to edition, so that the one-time pocket manual evolves into the two-volume multi-author tome and the library shelves groan under the load. This means that reading must be selective to be effective. I suggest that you will need at least one core textbook in each of your major subjects, and much of your reading will involve these. Sole reliance on the library for much-to-be-used textbooks is likely to lead to frustration as libraries have limited resources. Choose which book to purchase after reading the section on 'Using the library and buying books' in this guide.

In order to read effectively you have to be clear of your purpose. Ask yourself 'Why am I reading this?'. Ask yourself that question now of this book. Are you just scanning through for general interest or are you after detailed information? Your approach should vary with your purpose (Fig. 11.1). Let's look at an approach you might take to help with a serious piece of study. The important features of this widely recommended approach are summarized by SQR4 (Box 11.1).

Box 11.1 SQR4	
Scan	— For an overview
Question	— Decide what you want from your reading
Read	— An active process, looking for key material
Recall	— Periodically consider what you have covered
Review	— At the end, pull it all together
Relate	— Tie in with other topics – ***most important***

Imagine, for instance, the situation that last night you saw an elderly lady admitted to hospital, who had been found at home in an unheated flat. She was comatose and hypothermic, with a body temperature of 30°C. You now want to read up on the physiology of body temperature and its control. The Contents page or index

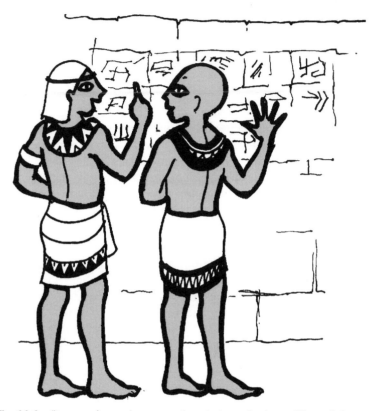

Fig. 11.1 'It warns of seven lean years, then starts on about something called 'global warming'.'

help you to find the right section of the physiology textbook you own. Apply the following approach:

1. Scan through the chapter to see what the subheadings are.

2. If there is a summary, read it through, identifying the main points and arguments that have been covered.

3. Ask yourself what you want to get from your reading.

4. Read the introductory paragraphs. They should set the scene.

5. Read the sections and subsections, actively identifying the main ideas in each. These ideas are often contained in the first (or sometimes last) sentence of the section or paragraph.

6. Look at any example. Make sure that you understand how it is related to the idea in that section.

7. Summarize periodically. Pause and list the main ideas in the section you have just read. Check that you have missed nothing out and that you understand the ideas.

8. Review the whole topic when you have finished it by scanning through your notes.

9. Relate what you have read to other areas of knowledge. For instance, on the science side you could relate changes in body temperature to what you know about how enzyme activity varies with temperature (biochemistry) or how the kidneys conserve fluid when the body is threatened by dehydration (other physiology). On the clinical side, you could look up how and why hypothermia management differs in the young and in the elderly, and think about the social aspects. Why was there no heating in the flat in the first place?

Note some things implicit in this approach to reading. First, the suggestion that you read a definite topic, not just 'the next chapter' or 'for 30 minutes'. Major textbooks are not meant to be read slavishly from cover to cover. However, scan through a new book for overviews of a subject and to familiarize yourself with the structure of the book. Also, note the emphasis on relating material in each section to other material. Research has shown that what is learnt and recalled is that most closely related to what the student already knows. That is, new material is most easily learnt when it can be slotted into a framework of previous knowledge. One of the great advantages of current changes to medical courses is the emphasis on an integrated approach to learning, and you will benefit from this particularly if you attend a medical school, such as Liverpool or Manchester, which bases much of its learning around clinical cases. If you had really dealt with the case outlined above I guarantee that you would never in the future be able to read about control of body temperature without recalling the case and its details, nor would you be able to have a discussion about resources and the care of the elderly without recalling the effect on health of having insufficient funds to provide heating. This power of integrated learning is why the 'Relate' activity of SQR4 is so important. (Those wanting to learn more about SQR4, or SQ3R from which it was adapted, should seek out Derek Rowntree's paperback *Learn to Study*, ISBN 0 7515 2088 8.)

Academic reading is active, not passive. It is hard work. You need a place where you can work comfortably and concentrate. Note-taking is a skill you will develop and use in both lectures (see that section of this guide) and private study. When reading, your notes should summarize the main ideas and examples so that you can understand the topic. Keep them brief. You are not attempting to copy out the textbook! Try to rephrase and summarize using your own words so that you are sure you understand. If you find difficulty understanding something try a different textbook – often you will find a different, more easily understandable, approach or a good explanatory diagram. Try using simple diagrams to help retention and form a pictorial relationship between different topics. If you learn by underlining or highlighting key sections of text as you read, do not forget the 'Recall', 'Review' and 'Relate' sections of the SQR4 technique. Also remember that library textbooks must not be so marked, only your own copies.

You will receive suggestions for further reading during lectures, tutorials etc. These come under a variety of names including Recommended reading, key references, Reading lists and general references. *Do not try to read everything.* Much of the suggested material will be of use if you wish to pursue a given area further, but there is not the time (nor do lecturers have the intention) for you to read it all. If you are unsure 'ask tutors and students from previous years what is required. If you find there is still too much, divide reading between two or three of you and grade material as essential, transmissible or not required. *Essential* is material which is so relevant that you feel your colleagues should read it first hand. *Transmissible* is material from which you can summarize the main points and pass them on, preferably with discussion. *Not required* is, well, not required. Often the latter references duplicate other reading while adding nothing, are really very peripheral or are out of date in a fast-moving field compared with other references. If the reading overload is great, a group of three or four working together may be able to halve the time needed to cover it. If using a group, allow a little time for everyone to get tuned in to what is required and what each other's needs are.

Pause at this point and use the SQR4 method on this section to see how well it works for you.

12

Good writing

A brief but ambitious title. This is a fairly extensive section dealing with an important area. Important not only because well written essays and reports will help you to gain good grades, but also because good written communication skills will be of use in much of your professional life.

There will be some advice and a few 'rules', but no magic formulae. We will be looking at one approach to writing an essay and some cautions about common pitfalls. I will give you some idea as to what I am looking for when marking an essay, and how it relates to a structure known as the 'SOLO' taxonomy. We will also look at the use of a structured marking sheet and the sometimes thorny issue of feedback. While this section concentrates on the writing of essays the fundamentals apply to other forms of writing, such as project reports, although these may have a slightly different and more formalized structure (Fig. 12.1).

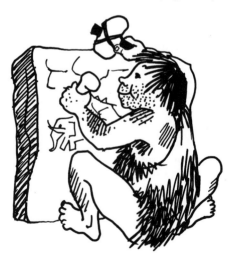

Fig. 12.1 Good writing requires planning and time.

Let's look first at why we ask you to write essays. Foremost we want you to develop certain skills and abilities. First among these is the ability to construct a balanced, coherent argument using available evidence. Occasionally, the topic requires a largely factual account but usually we are interested in your own assessments and views, informed by the writings and opinions of others. The gathering and evaluation of evidence is therefore one of the most important stages of writing. Essays are not generally being used to test the extent of your factual knowledge because multiple-choice and short-answer questions are better suited to this role.

Your experience in writing essays will vary enormously. If you are already a graduate experienced in essay and report writing, you may wish just to skim through this section to see if there are any additional tips to pick up. If you are entering medical school with A levels in chemistry, physics and maths, detailed study is likely to be worthwhile as essays are unlikely to have featured heavily in your recent studies. If you entered medical school having studied subjects such as English or psychology at A level, or via a baccalaureate, you are likely to be somewhere in between. Again, fairly detailed study should prove worthwhile.

PLANNING AN ESSAY

We will consider this in sections in the order I suggest you use (see Box 12.1).

Box 12.1 Stages in planning an essay
(Preliminaries)
Title
Thoughts
Outline
Literature
First draft
(Pause)
Second draft
(Pause)
Essay
(Submission)

Before reading on look carefully at the order in Box 12.1 from title to essay. Is there anything that surprises you?

Preliminaries

There are certain preliminaries about which you must be clear. How long is the essay to be? What is the submission date? Is it acceptable as a handwritten essay or does it have to be printed?

Length usually has some flexibility. I take no exception to stipulated length plus or minus 10%. If there are many references, an appendix, tables or diagrams, check to see whether they are to be included in the overall length. References, and essential tables and diagrams, may well be exempt. On the other hand an appendix may have to be counted – otherwise it can be used as a device to avoid having to stick to length (Fig. 12.2). If you feel you can 'cover the topic' in well under the required length, then think again very carefully. Ask yourself if you have tackled the topic to the

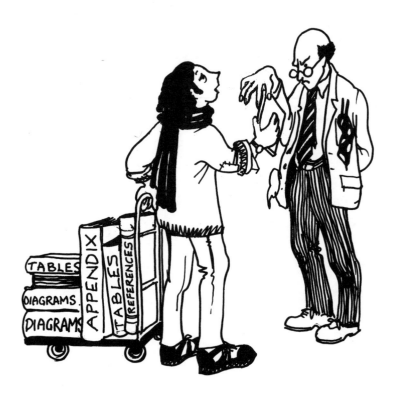

Fig. 12.2 'Yes, the essay itself is only 3000 words as required.'

depth and breadth required. Read the section on SOLO taxonomy (below) and have a brainstorming session with fellow students before deciding for certain that your brevity is appropriate.

Unlike length, the submission date is usually negotiable in only one direction. You can hand work in before the due date but not afterwards. Punctuality of this type is important in professional life. Do not rely on a kind tutor – the previously most approachable tutor can turn to steel at requests for extensions. If you have a genuine reason for difficulty in meeting a submission date, discuss it with your tutor as far in advance as possible. Good reasons are major illness of self (or a relative) or a bereavement, but don't claim the death of your Auntie May too often as it strains credibility (Fig. 12.3). Reasons such as having lost your notes or having been on a week's tour with the University Hockey Club will not be welcomed. You are expected to organize your own resources and time.

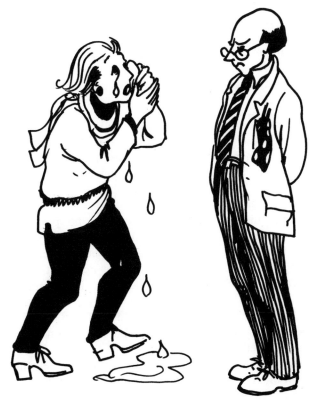

Fig. 12.3 '...and what is it to be for Auntie May this time – a burial or a cremation?'

Nowadays, on many courses there is a stipulation that written work should be printed rather than handwritten. In practice this means using a word processor. You may feel this is unfair if you write in a beautiful rounded script, but few do and a difficult-to-read script can double of treble marking time. Poorly legible scripts also lose marks. This is not necessarily because of any deliberate deduction by the marker. It is simply because following an argument is more difficult if you have to concentrate on deciphering hieroglyphs at the same time.

The title

Usually you will be given a title. Titles vary in their specificity. Look at the following list:

- Describe neuronal conduction in the squid nerve axon.
- Outline the stages of Krebs' cycle.
- Critically review factors involved in a shift of health care to the primary sector.
- 'Androgens should be available to athletes as over-the counter drugs.' Discuss.
- A famous physician said 'Diagnosis is everything.' Is this view valid?

The first two titles, about squid axons and Krebs' cycle, seem to be seeking a largely factual account to test a knowledge base. As noted above, as there are other ways to test a knowledge base this type of essay title is becoming less common. Detailed knowledge of these specific topics is of questionable value in a modern medical curriculum in any event.

Look at the third title. This is more open to interpretation with respect to scope. Are we talking only about the UK here, or including changes in developing countries which are realizing that centralized, expensive medical services are not what they most need? Note that we are not being asked to *list* or *enumerate* factors but to *review critically*. We are required not only to survey the topic but to assess the value of the factors we mention, stating our own judgement as to their validity and also stating on what that judgement is based.

The essay about androgens has the feel of an essay set when this topic was in the news. *Discuss* again means critical analysis and the evaluation of evidence for and against the thesis. Your views and conclusions may well differ from mine but if we both wrote on the topic we would expect to be marked on the cogency of our arguments, not on whether our views matched those of the marker. The writer has the right to expect objectivity from the marker of such a topic.

The final title, about the statement 'Diagnosis is everything', requires the same analytical treatment as the previous two. Just because a statement raises your blood pressure (as this does mine, as it is so against all the principles of holistic care), this is not a reason for abandoning all dispassionate objectivity when writing about it! For instance, you could set the statement in the context of the limited treatment and management options available at the time is was made, a small redeeming factor.

Finally, what if you have not been given a title? You will have been given some general topic area, such as 'Write a 3000-word essay on some topic related to medical education, primary health care, a major infectious disease, etc.'. Beware of choosing too broad an area. While initially this may seem an easy option there are several problems, of which you rapidly become aware. The breadth means that depth is impossible to achieve and you drop into descriptive mode, which will neither gain high grades nor usefully develop your writing skills. You will be overwhelmed by 'relevant' references as soon as you try to look up information. If you find the chosen topic is too broad after initial thoughts and a look at the literature, then re-focus at that stage and *change the title appropriately*. Do not wait until your perusal of the second draft, 3 days before the deadline. Gibbon's *The Decline and Fall of the Roman Empire* extends to 1700 pages – better in an essay to limit yourself to Attila the Hun's invasion of Gaul rather than try to produce a condensed version of the whole.

Thoughts and outline

The next two stages are linked. First, you need to jot down your thoughts on the topic. Do not try to restrict these at this stage. I use either a simple list with no ordering or a mind-map. For a mind-map you put the topic at the centre of the page and then any thoughts on the topic around it in a radiating pattern. These 'thoughts' may have related thoughts running out from them. (Before reading further, take a break for 5 minutes and construct a first list or mind-map on the title 'Androgens should be available to athletes as over-the-counter drugs'. Discuss.) Keep the list or mind-map handy in the kitchen of your flat or in your room and add more ideas to it over the next couple of days. Think about allowing your flat-mates to add ideas as well – especially valuable if they are not themselves medics. Link up any associated ideas, put question marks by any you think are not relevant on a second look and asterisk those you think are particularly good. The second stage is to construct some sort of order from your ideas to get across the arguments that you want to make. Thirty or forty minutes is then usually enough to plan a rough outline of the essay.

Some of my thoughts about the 'androgens and athletes', essay are shown below:

- ?Evidence of performance benefit
- Malignancy risk
- 'Sportsmanship' definition
- Gain from being sponsored
- Cost
- Fairness in sport
- Behavioural change
  — Aggression
  — Family damage
- Physical damage
  — ?Sexual function
  — ?Heart
- Use of indirect androgen stimulants
- ?Benefit in all sports or just energy sports
  — ?Athletics, rowing but not cricket.

I expect you had some different ideas, but also some that overlap with mine. *Note that at this stage you have not been to seek out relevant literature.* This is where the sequence I recommend differs from that commonly given in guides about study skills. Generally they recommend looking up the literature as the first stage after being given the title.

The literature

I suggest that only now do you look at the literature. I recommend this sequence for two reasons. First, if you go to the literature and read a couple of review articles, you are far less likely to adopt an original approach or use original arguments. Second, if you start off by using information sources like Medline and the World Wide Web (WWW) you are likely to end up with hundreds or thousands of articles to look at. With the approach recommended it is easier to conduct a more focused and precise search, as you know the questions which you are seeking evidence to answer. Your search may eventually lead you to include areas not on your mind-map. You may discard other areas that initially looked promising. But you will not be in the position of having an unfocused approach with hundreds of articles to read, and of not knowing when you can stop reading and move on to the next important stage, the first draft.

First draft–Pause–Second draft

For the first draft you need to find a quiet hour or two. The draft does not contain the full text or all the detail. It provides the shape of the introduction, the body of the essay and the main conclusions. The body of the essay will be a linked sequence of arguments, with examples, references and reservations where necessary, that supports the major points that you decided in your outline to make. Your conclusion will follow naturally from these without introducing new material. *Pause.* Put the draft aside for a day or two and then re-read it. Is it logical and interrelated? Have you kept to the topic? Have you said what you want to say? If the answers are yes, yes and yes then prepare a fuller second draft before the final paper. *Pause* again if there is time and leave the second draft aside for a week, then re-read it. Does it still look as good? Think about the written style as well as the content. Still OK? Pass it over to a fellow student for constructive criticism. He/she will often pick up points which are unclear to them, although readily understood by you because of your greater background reading in the area. These need clarification. Check that the draft is of the right length.

Final essay

The final essay needs the amendments to the second draft to be incorporated. Take special care that no new errors are introduced. This is particularly easy to do when using cut-and-paste on a word processor, as parts of sentences can be left behind or moved by accident. Check that any references are correct and that they are in a standard format. Check that everything you wanted to say has been said. Check that you are happy with the layout. Check that the essay has your name and contact details on the front sheet. Run it through a spell-checker. There is no excuse for dozens of spelling errors in a word-processed essay.

Submission

This will of course be on time. If submitting a printed version, you will keep a photocopy or second printed version in case the first is lost in the post or by the marker. If submitting on disk you will keep a copy disk. You will also check the disk to be submitted, to see that it carries no virus. Virus-checkers will be available on your university network or on disk from the university computing service. If submitting electronically, you will keep a safe copy and will not submit with a file name such as 'essay. doc'. This would be instantly overwritten by each of the next 30 students who submits under the same file name. This is the only time when it can be an advantage to submit late and last!

Summary

Again, in summary:

Title – Thoughts – Outline – Literature – First draft – Pause – Second draft – Pause – Essay

An essay or project report requires a lot of forward planning. Note that compared with those who are writing by hand, those using a word processor may be slower at the first draft but will probably be a lot faster at turning the second draft into the final paper.

WRITING STYLE

We will move on to look at some aspects of writing style, concentrating on grammatical considerations, layout and finally on some general considerations.

Grammar

A simple writing style aids clarity. Use simple words, simple sentences and simple paragraphs, even for complex ideas. By the use of simple words I mean use much the same vocabulary as you would if you were speaking to a colleague on the same topic. This does not mean including 'uhms' and 'ahs' or slang expressions in the text, but it does mean avoiding unnecessarily complex words. If you would say 'We changed over the left and rights leads' you need not write 'The dextral and sinistral leads were transposed'. Read your essay aloud. Are there any words or phrases which would not be understood by any fellow students whose first language is not English? If so, try to simplify them. At times you will, of course, be using technical language. You would write '...the four quadrants of the abdomen...' and not '...the compass points of the tummy...'.

A simple sentence contains one idea and not more than one subordinate clause. On the whole use simple sentences. If you read a sentence and it is not at once clear which part of the sentence is related to which other part of the sentence then it needs rewriting. Thus this last sentence is unclear: what does 'it' in 'it needs rewriting' refer to? Do I mean the whole sentence or specifically the part of the sentence whose relationship to the whole sentence is unclear? Changing 'it' to 'the whole sentence' clarifies things. Often, rewriting a long sentence to increase clarity involves splitting the sentence into two. Remember, a sentence contains a subject and a verb. As a rule write in sentences, and if you break this rule do so consciously. As the eagle-eyed among you will already have noticed, the first 'sentence' of this whole chapter is not a sentence. (It is 'A brief but ambitious title.'.)

Limit the use of clichés in your writing. A cliché is an overused literary phase. Examples are 'eagle-eyed' (used above), 'on top of the world' and 'putting all your eggs in one basket'. Similarly, limit your use of metaphors. A metaphor is the application of a name or descriptive term to an object to which it is not literally applicable, for example '...prisoners were guinea pigs...'. In particular avoid mixed metaphors, which can conjure up more than one image. One of my students, writing about change in medical education, wrote '...we are all guinea pigs on the roller-coaster of medical education...'. The image was delightful, but distracted from the argument in the text (Fig. 12.4).

Paragraphs should have one theme. This theme is generally outlined in the first sentence of the paragraph. The rest of the paragraph expands on the theme. Having been given the theme, the reader knows what to look for in the rest of the paragraph. The theme often links with the previous paragraph, or the final sentence of the previous paragraph forms the link with the next. For example, 'The above arguments about the economic causes of unemployment in the 1920s are persuasive but now let us move on to a second theme, the social consequences of that unemploy-ment.'. These links are of vital importance in the flow of your essay – they make your reader want to read on from one section to the next and from one page to the next.

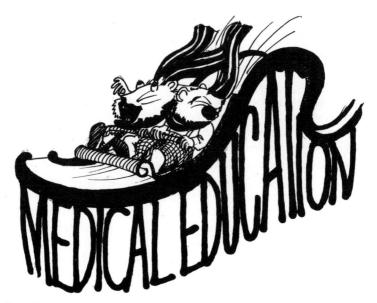

Fig. 12.4 Mixed metaphors: 'We are all guinea pigs on the roller-coaster of medical education.'

Consider the overall text difficulty. Major word processors such as Microsoft Word and WordPerfect have grammar-checkers which include an index, such as the Flesch Reading Ease Score (FRES), which shows how difficult a piece of text is to read. Scores in the 40s represent text which is 'fairly difficult', those in the 50s 'fairly easy' and those in the 60s and 70s 'easy'. The calculation is based on things such as sentence length and syllables per word. Flesch himself acknowledged that many short sentences could become dull to read. He recommended varying the sentence length and averaging about 17 words per sentence. This chapter has a Flesch score of 61 and an average sentence length of 15 words. You can find out more about the FRES, and related Fog Index, using your newly developed WWW searching skills.

Layout

Good layout helps your reader. Try to make the overall appearance of the page attractive. Leave adequate margins for your tutor's comments and use only one side of the paper. Leave a blank between sections and consider leaving one between paragraphs.

Headings and subheadings can be underlined or, preferably, emboldened if using a word processor. Use a common standard font such as Arial or Times New Roman, and avoid the exotic fonts from Aardvark to Zurich Calligraphic. In a long essay, Times Roman is arguably more cursive to the eye than Arial. Use a font size which will not remind the marker of his/her progressively developing middle-age myopia. This means using a font size of no less than 10-point, and preferably 12-point. Format the text so that it is left-justified rather than fully-justified. Although full justification gives straight left and right margins it gives odd text spacing and can leave rivers of space flowing down the page from top to bottom.

The essay title should be at the top of the page along with your name and contact details so that the essay can be returned or discussed. In a substantial formal essay these details may go on a separate front sheet.

General considerations

There are several general considerations. The essay will be written with an overall structure. The most common structure involves an introduction to set the context, followed by the body of the essay and then the conclusion or summary. The body of the essay contains a linked sequence of arguments, each of which may itself be divided into introduction, body and summary.

Essays often contain quotations from published papers or textbooks. A word of caution. *Quotations must always be clearly indicated in your essay by enclosure in quotation marks.* It is often helpful also to put the quotation in italics to clearly distinguish it from your own text. Quotations must be accurate and words should not be changed. If part of a quote is omitted, this is indicated by three dots (...) at the appropriate point in the text. If you introduce additional words for clarification, enclose them in square brackets: '...despite repeated questions he [Prime Minister] refused to confirm the Chancellor's comments...'. This device clarifies that the 'he' in the quote refers to the Prime Minister. Quotations should be referenced. Using text without indicating it is not your own is termed *plagiarism*. It is a hanging offence. This must be stressed. Academics have lost their reputations and careers because of plagiarism. Students have failed their finals. Using other students' work, even if not published, is similarly regarded as plagiarism and attracts the same penalties. In the context of a medical course quotations should in any case be used sparingly and to illustrate a specific point, and not used extensively.

ASSESSING ESSAYS

Writing essays is difficult. So is assessing the quality of essays. Many markers of essays do not compare their approach to those of their colleagues. They say things like 'Well, it was clearly worth an Upper Second, not a First', but they are unable to define why. There are several approaches to making assessment more reliable. We will look at two. One is based on a method known as the SOLO taxonomy. The other, which we will consider first, is to use a structured marking sheet.

Structured marking sheets

The Leeds structured marking sheet allocates marks for each of a number of categories on a 0–10 or 0–5 scale. The essay is marked twice: once by a member of staff, who also adds comments, and once by the student. The student knows what criteria are to be used to mark the essay before it is written, and this itself helps to improve his/her writing. If the marks given by student and tutor are close or the tutor's mark is higher, then the student gets the higher mark. If opinions differ there is a set adjudication system. Marks are given in each of three areas, these being *content* (0–10), *interpretation* (0–10) and *presentation* (0–5). The features we consider are shown in Boxes 12.2, 12.3 and 12.4. The lower end of each scale represents the opposite criterion. Thus, 'Critical analysis of cited papers (10)' would be complemented by 'Uncritical, little analysis or evaluation (0)'.

Box 12.2 Essay content (0–10 scale)

Clear, referenced introduction
Comprehensive, relevant literature review
Sufficient depth of key references
Conclusions justified by evidence

Box 12.3 Essay interpretation (0–10 scale)

Critical analysis of cited papers
Logically presented, well focused
Evidence of originality
Good discussion of possible clinical implications

Box 12.4 Essay presentation (0–5 scale)

Clear layout with appropriate headings, diagrams and tables
Approximately required length
Sentences grammatical/spelling correct
References correctly cited in text and reference list

The advantage of structured marking is that there is some objectivity, by its nature there is a degree of feedback and students learn to assess their own work. One disadvantage is that the schema may not be appropriate for some essays, for instance an essay not considering clinical implications and with no need for tables or diagrams might suffer unfairly. Also, the marks are given for the *process* of writing the essay. At least some argue that in this schema, insufficient regard is given to content. Others argue that it is process we are primarily aiming to encourage.

SOLO taxonomy

Let us look at a more general and in some ways less structured method of grading an essay. This method is based on the *SOLO taxonomy*, a taxonomy devised by an educationalist, Professor John Biggs.

The ideas in this small section may seem complex. Persevere! An understanding of the five different levels involved in the SOLO taxonomy will enable you to improve your marks in essays and projects considerably. Remember that the way you write an essay not only reflects your knowledge of a particular subject, but beyond this can show how well you can analyze a topic and integrate it with other areas of thought or knowledge. At university it is this higher level of understanding in which we are most interested. It is a reflection of the quality of the learning outcome and is summarized in the SOLO taxonomy, where 'SOLO' stands for 'Structures of the Observed Learning Outcome'.

There are five SOLO levels (see Box 12.5).

Box 12.5   SOLO levels

1. **Prestructural** = Ignorance!

2. **Unistructural** = Single correct and relevant item of content

3. **Multistructural** = Several relevant items, but considered independently in the essay rather than being related

4. **Relational** = Relevant items related into an overall structure and argument, rather than being listed

5. **Extended abstract** = Items are not only related into a structure but if relevant are related to other wider domains of knowledge, showing an understanding of 'the questions behind the question'

Take a more concrete example. A class is asked to write an essay on the control of blood pressure. Pause to jot down what you would include, and how you would relate the material, before reading on.

Those with *unistructural* approach address the topic in terms of control of the systolic and diastolic blood pressure.

Those with a *multistructural* approach have additional sections, dealing with the cerebral circulation, the renal and visceral circulation and the blood supply to the heart. But while they are addressed, they are addressed as separate items. Knowledge of the one is not used to inform that of the other.

The *relational* approach would consider the mechanisms of control of each circulation, compare and contrast the different problems they face and how they solve the problems that arise under different circumstances.

The *extended abstract* approach might in addition take the overview that what we are really considering is the homeostasis of body systems, of which this is one example. While consideration is mainly related to *Homo sapiens*, other mammals face problems peculiar to themselves and must have adopted additional coping mechanisms. For instance, how does the giraffe maintain cerebral perfusion when moving from drinking to upright posture (Fig. 12.5)?

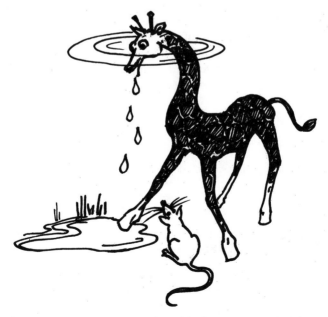

Fig. 12.5 Mouse: 'Dizzy after a drink you say? Can't say I've ever noticed that problem.'

A useful exercise is to take a few topics and sketch an outline of content at the various levels of approach. Look at a few old essays and see at what level they were written. How easy would it have been to move up a level?

In broad terms, in degree assessments the first class honours students take the Extended abstract approach and those achieving upper seconds take the Relational approach, whereas those achieving lower seconds rarely extent beyond the Multistructural approach. If you understand the levels it is relatively easy to make the transition from level 2 to level 3 and from level 3 to level 4. It is rather more difficult to make the transition from level 4 to level 5. I would not expect any of you to remain at level 2.

Feedback

Finally, a brief look at what you can expect by way of feedback. Whatever marking scheme is used it is vital that you receive feedback, and that it is in a form that helps you to improve your writing. This means that you need to seek specific comments and not generalities. A comment such as 'A modest effort overall' is not particularly useful. Comments of more use might be 'An interesting idea, but looking at this section again can you offer any alternative explanation which could lead to a different conclusion?' or 'If you put in a first sentence to say what was to be covered in this section, do you think it would be clearer for the reader?'. Comments on written work need to be made within a reasonable time or they lose their impact as you have moved on in the course. However, marking 200+ essays conscientiously is a huge workload and a satisfactory compromise may be difficult to reach. If looking at the *process* of writing, group feedback highlighting major common strengths and problems may prove to be the best solution. The same approach can be used to cover *content* if there is a limited range of essay titles. Using a structured assessment form, as discussed above, gets over some of the problems, but not all.

SUMMARY

In summary, enjoy writing and write to inform and learn. It is common that in any substantial essay you will develop knowledge in advance of not only your fellow students but also some of your tutors. More importantly, you will have the joy of the sudden flashes of insight that you get when evidence combines and leads to an unexpected conclusion. A colleague once told me that she preferred defending a minority position rather than the accepted view because of the understanding that it gave her that when she was in the majority she might nevertheless be wrong. Original writing gives you the opportunity to realize that this can indeed be the case. After all, we now know that the earth is not flat.

Using the library and buying books

'*Books must follow sciences and not sciences books.*'

(Francis Bacon, 1561–1626)

USING THE LIBRARY

While this proposition is undoubtedly true, in order to learn both basic science and clinical medicine we must certainly 'follow' (in the sense of 'understand') books. Efficient use of the medical school library is essential if you are both to write and read effectively in the way outlined in previous chapters. Your main medical school library will contain tens of thousands of books and journals, and its very size can seem daunting at first. However, its major sections and roles in student life are easily understood. Whilst the exact layout of libraries does of course vary most are divided into similar sections as described below and have similar arrangements for borrowing books and periodicals.

You will use the library for three main purposes: quiet study, looking up material in journals or in electronic reference sources, and borrowing or consulting textbooks. To enter and use the library you will need a valid user's ticket, which in some schools is incorporated into the student card. Frequently it will be an electronic or bar-coded swipe card, used to open a barrier.

The library will have three main sections. These are for current periodicals, bound periodicals and textbooks.

Periodicals

Current periodicals and bound periodicals are each arranged alphabetically by title. At the end of each bay there is a notice saying which range of journals is contained in that bay (e.g. 'Exp

Brain Res to J Community Psychol'). The current periodicals section contains the latest edition of each periodical and frequently the last few issues, typically for the current volume. The bound periodicals section contains previous volumes of each journal, and usually the different sections of the journal which make up the volume are bound together. Within the bound periodicals section the volumes of any one title are arranged chronologically, as you would expect.

Try looking up a reference. References are papers referred to by the writer of a paper in the text of his/her paper. Visit the library, pick a current journal and flick through to the list of references at the end of a paper. You will see something like:

Palenicek J G, Graham N M H, He Y H et al 1995 Weight loss prior to clinical AIDS as a predictor of survival. J Acquir Immune Defic Syndr 10: 366

The format may differ slightly but usually includes authors, title of paper, journal title, volume number, first and last page numbers and year of publication. Here the publication year is 1995, journal volume is 10 and first page number is 366. In this case the last page number is not included. Three authors are identified by name and the others are included in the all-encompassing 'el al', meaning 'and other authors'. These will be listed on the actual paper but not when referenced, to save space. This is a common practice with multiple authors. Choose a reference, preferably from the last 10 years, from the list in your journal and see if you can hunt it down. The latest issue of a journal often has to be read in the library, but earlier issues and bound journals can generally be taken out on overnight loan. Often in the area where the journals are kept are cubicles and desks. Use these for quiet study. You may bring your own books into the library to work with, as well as using the library's.

Textbooks

The medical textbooks are filed in a section of the library separately from the bound journals, and arranged rather differently. They are collected in different sections according to subject and classmark. For instance, books on the respiratory system have the classmark WF, and those on physiology have QT. The letters themselves (WF, QT) have no logical meaning other than to professional librarians and are best just accepted as being the letters used for a given subject. Classes are indicated at the ends of bays, and may be further subdivided. For example:

QT   Physiology

104–172   Human physiology

180–275   Physiology/Sports medicine/Hygiene

Guyton's *'Textbook of Physiology'* is a popular book. It will be filed alphabetically by author in this section, labelled QT 104 GUY – 'GUY' being the first three letters of the author's surname.

Most textbooks may be borrowed from the library for a more generous period than is the case with periodicals, but it will vary from a few days to a few weeks depending on the library. Certain books, which are heavily used, will be on overnight loan and some may form part of a counter collection, for use only in the library for a few hours. These books are available from the counter on request and not filed on the general shelves. This group often comprises books referenced by a lecturer at some specific point in the course, or textbooks needed by many students to complete a project. The borrowers of books (and periodicals) are subject to fines if the items are kept beyond their return date. Fines can quickly become substantial, so keep an eye on return dates. Books are usually electronically tagged and have to be cleared by the librarian at the check-out desk before they are taken from the library, or an alarm goes off as you cross the exit. If it sounds then blush, go back to get the book cleared and be more careful in future.

Your search for a textbook is helped by use of the *On-line Public Catalogue* (OPC) or equivalent. This is a computerized catalogue telling you what journals and books are taken by the library and under what classmark the books are to be found. By following a series of simple instructions on the screen you can search the catalogue by things such as subject area, author or title. If the book or journal is held in a university library other than the main medical library, it will often tell you this too.

Other services

The library also provides many other services to help you in your studies. You will be able to photocopy a paper (although the page cost is low, it quickly mounts up) or perform an in-depth search on a subject using bibliographies held in databases on the computer network. This is not difficult and very valuable during project work. The most commonly consulted database is probably Medline, which contains abstracts of millions of medical papers published over the last 20 years or so. Search is by topic, key word, author, etc. and is usually straightforward. However, ask the library if they are running training sessions, as making complex searches with a high 'hit' rate of relevant papers takes some skill. Relevant abstracts found in searches may be viewed on screen, printed out or saved to disk. Often you will find a section in the abstract called 'Local information' or the equivalent. This tells you whether the journal is held in the medical library or in another university library, or if it will have to be obtained from an outside source if you want to study the full paper. The cost of obtaining a reference and the time to acquire it increase progressively the further the source is from the home library. Many doctors use little other than Medline but explore other databases, especially the Cochrane Library and CINAHL (Cumulative Index to Nursing and Allied Health Literature) databases. The Cochrane Library database contains systematic up-to-date reviews on health care and information on randomized controlled trials. You want to know what is the best treatment for an irregular heartbeat after a transient stroke? It's there. All the information you need, studied and evaluated by someone else. A great help. The CINAHL database contains a different spectrum of information and research and is complementary to Medline but more orientated to work from nursing and the allied professions. While these databases will almost certainly be available in the library, they may be accessible over the university network as well.

You will be given a guided tour of the library soon after you start at medical school. Much of the above will be explained to you and you will probably be supplied with leaflets about library services, opening times and how to borrow books. There are also many other printed leaflets available, telling you things such as how to obtain a reference, photocopy or use the on-line public catalogue to find out if a book you want is in stock.

In some corner of the library will be serried ranks of bound volumes of *Index Medicus*, a different colour for each year and each year occupying several feet of shelf space. This is the paper version of the type of information held in Medline. It allows you to look up the titles and journal locations of relevant papers on a given topic, but contains no abstracts. With the advent of electronic databases *Index Medicus* is as outdated as the quill pen and the abacus. Steer clear of it.

Will you make mistakes, fail to find references which are there and not know how to tackle a particulars search you want? Certainly, and the library staff, who are expert in such things, will be pleased to help you out and explain where you are going wrong so you will manage more easily the next time.

BUYING BOOKS

For personal study you almost certainly need at least one core textbook in each of the major subjects and in some other areas. Thus, starting a medical firm you need not only a textbook on medicine but also one on the clinical history and examination. The library will not contain enough copies of standard textbooks to meet your need, nor is it likely to have sufficiently long or 'convenient' opening hours. Libraries seem unable to meet the needs of those students who want an evening out and then strong coffee and a couple of hours' work around midnight.

The major popular undergraduate textbooks are sold in substantial numbers and retain their market position over many editions. As the field is competitive, they are keenly priced and represent good value. Even a newcomer will be priced to match the market. School courses tend to work from a specified set book, but for most university courses you have greater freedom of choice. So you need to purchase, but how do you decide which book to buy and from where should you buy it?

Choosing

First, talk to last year's students. Hear what they have to say about the various books in the relevant subject, be it anatomy, surgery or statistics. Was the coverage excessive or insufficient? Was it up to date? Was the course keyed to that textbook, another or none? Second, go to the library and spend some time with the books. You will not of course understand the whole content, but try to get a 'feel' for a book. Is the text style readable and are the illustrations clear? Is the text clearly subdivided into sections with subheadings, or are you faced with a monotonous sea of print? Does each chapter/ section have a summary of what it contains or an introductory section on what is to be covered? Dip into an early section and look at the sentence and paragraph lengths. It can be difficult to work from textbooks which contain multiple ideas in complex sentences running to many lines. Ask yourself *'Would I enjoy working from this book?'*. Third, talk to those giving the particular course and check that the book you propose to purchase is suitable and that the course does not require students to work from a given textbook.

You will find that few books take an integrated approach to medical education – most are discipline-specific. While the approach suggested in *Tomorrow's Doctors* has far from fully filtered down to authors, basic science textbooks increasingly highlight clinical examples and clinical textbooks increasingly include sections on basic science. You may find that you require more than one textbook to match your needs for a specific course. For instance, on a medical firm you may find you like to work from a standard medical textbook which takes a disease-orientated approach, along with a second book which takes a case-based or symptom-based approach.

Purchasing

There are two main ways you can purchase books – new and second-hand. Most university towns, and some others, have many excellent bookshops and there may also be a bookshop on campus. Currently, there is little point in shopping around because usually the price of new textbooks does not vary between different shops. However, check to see whether there is a cheaper paperback version available if you see only a hardback version. Check before purchasing that a new edition of the book is not about to appear. While book-shops tend to offer each textbook at about the same price, a number of retailers now sell books over the Internet, which may enable you to save a little even after postage costs. Do not buy just from having seen a flyer which is attractive. They all are. Make sure that you see the book itself to check that it suits you.

Students in later years of their course frequently sell books that they used in the earlier parts, especially when they progress from the second to the third year – the old (but now lessening) preclinical/ clinical divide. These second-hand books may represent good value for money, saving perhaps 50% of the cost of a brand-new textbook. Be a little circumspect. Form an independent judgement on the suitability of the book for the course and for yourself, as discussed above. Don't purchase a 'bargain' on the sole recom-mendation of the seller. Expect a second-hand book to have signs of having been well used. If it is 'as new', is it really likely to have been suitable for the course? Check which edition you are buying and ask yourself whether it is likely to be sufficiently up to date. Some subjects advance rapidly, e.g. molecular biology, and a 4-year-old textbook may be hopelessly out of date, whereas in other subjects progress is not as fast, e.g. undergraduate anatomy, and a textbook may change little over a 5–10-year period. If a textbook appears to be other than the latest or penultimate edition don't buy it. Publishers normally reprint to generate further copies, and go to the expense of a new edition only in order to incorporate new material and delete that which is outdated.

14

Tutorials and small group work

You will meet several types of small group work, including laboratory work, project work, clinical bedside teaching and possibly anatomical dissection. Tutorials fall into and overlap with this family. Here I am using the term 'tutorial' particularly to cover those sessions which involve a tutor, generally with some specialist knowledge, and a small number of students talking through a topic for 30–90 minutes. The number of students varies, but is commonly between two and eight. It is generally necessary to split groups of more than eight students into subgroups for discussion. When they work well, tutorials can be some of the most stimulating sessions that you can have; when they work badly they can degenerate into mini-lectures by the tutor or dialogues between the tutor and one student, the rest taking no part. Below we will look at how we can make tutorials run productively, and then move on to look briefly at laboratory-based work.

TUTORIALS

Tutorials can have a variety of formats, for example topic clarification, case study/problem-solving, student presentation and discussion (e.g. ethical dilemma). They can also have a variety of goals (see Box 14.1). For instance, tutorials can promote discussion, clarify a difficult topic and provide a chance to go into a topic in more depth than is possible in a lecture. They give you the chance to express your views and knowledge as well as learning the skill of listening to others. At a social level, they allow more personal contact with other students and your tutors, reducing isolation and making it easier to seek help or guidance at other times.

The tutorial group composition may be fixed or variable. When the focus is on topic clarification the composition will probably be variable, involving just those students who are having difficulty

Box 14.1   Goals of tutorials

The development of:

- problem-solving skills
- attitudinal change
- group working skills
- debating/discussion skills
- leadership skills
- time management skills
- social interaction.

with the topic. Clearly, if a large proportion of the class is having difficulty a large group teaching session of some form is likely to be used in preference. For most other purposes, a fixed group has advantages. This is because it takes time for any group of individuals to get to the point at which they are working together productively. It is helpful to understand the four stages that small groups usually go through. These are sometimes described as *forming*, *storming*, *norming* and *performing*.

At the *forming* stage, the individuals have yet to get to know each other. Characteristics include tentativeness and hesitancy. The focus is not on the task but on developing relationships within the group. Usually participation is uneven, anxiety levels are high and nonproductive silences are common. Most do not find this stage enjoyable.

During the *storming* stage, the group members start to discuss how they are going to operate, shifting allegiances develop, differences of approach and value become evident and personalities clash.

In the *norming* stage, ground rules are worked out and you decide how you are going to tackle the task. The focus shifts from group dynamics to the task.

Finally, during the *performing* stage, the group tackles the task productively and its members often find great enjoyment in working as a group and in the support given and received by other members. Non-group members may be seen as 'outsiders' and not welcomed. Different members of the group adopt different roles to contribute to a common solution. Members feel valued by the group.

An awareness that the forming and storming stages are often necessary before groups can begin to function truly productively will help you if you are not used to group work, in which case these stages can seem rather frightening. A good tutor will allow these stages to happen, while placing some limit on them so that the group progresses and does not break up. A mark of the tutor's success may be that in later sessions, the cohesion of the student group means that the tutor is no longer really welcomed as a participant! If the early stages do not take place, there is a risk of storming taking place later and the task not being completed.

Successful tutorials require the *3Ps*. These are *Planning*, *Preparation* and *Participation*. For each of these three activities there is dual responsibility – that of the tutor and that of the student.

Planning involves knowing what is to be covered in advance. You must discuss this with your tutor and fellow students. Tutorials are generally flexible and, with advance planning, the content should reflect your own and your fellow students' needs. Without a knowledge of what is planned, preparation is impossible.

Preparation will vary. It may be reading up on a lecture or clinical topic, or spending a few minutes sorting out your views on an ethical issue. It may be just deciding what questions you want discussed and what potential answers you can suggest.

Participation by students is the third requirement of a successful tutorial. Students are often reluctant to speak. The tutor's problem is often the reverse. He/she has to avoid filling the void of silence by turning the whole thing into a mini-lecture. Speaking up in a group may seem difficult at first, but your tutor understands this and you will have the support of your fellow students too. There is the fear that you might show yourself up, or you may feel that you have nothing to add. Don't be too reticent about speaking up. The best discussions are not made up of a series of brilliant, totally original statements but by building up step by step. Ask for clarification, or pull together or contrast the suggestions that have gone before. Talk to the group, not back and forth to the tutor, and help bring others in by asking what they think. Participation is far easier when you are part of a stable tutorial group which has gone through the stages of group formation described above. The physical environment in which the tutorial takes place can have a profound effect on its success or otherwise, and it is worth spending a little time to ensure that this is right (Fig. 14.1).

Traditionally and ideally, tutorial groups comprise eight or less students, but with growing numbers of students and decreasing numbers of tutors the size of tutorial groups is growing. Because the opportunity to contribute is such a valuable part of the tutorial process, various ways are used to ensure that students will continue to be able to participate. Three common ways you will meet are *brainstorming*, *dyads* and *snowballs*.

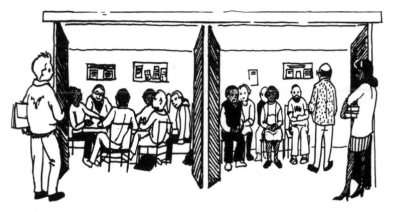

Fig. 14.1 a   John: 'Enjoy the debate.'   **b**   Mary: 'Waste of time, a mini-lecture.'

Brainstorming is used to generate ideas, which are later sorted and evaluated for their relevance to a particular problem. For instance, in a group considering how to improve tutorials, members would each suggest the first idea that came into their head. These would all be listed without comment or evaluation and form the basis for later work. For example, suggestions could be 'not on Friday afternoons', 'alter seating', 'students/tutors decide topic jointly', 'tea and cakes'. Students contribute in turn or at random.

In *dyads*, students break up into pairs and work on the problem. If the form of the problem means that each has to explain something to the other and then listen to an explanation in turn, even the shy contribute and the overly loquacious must listen.

In a *snowball* approach, the group breaks up into subgroups of pairs or fours to tackle the problem and these then coalesce into groups of, say, eight before reporting back to the full group of, say, thirty-two. If you are threatened with a mini-lecture because of student numbers when the topic is better suited to group work, then suggest a snowball approach.

Tutorials are for the benefit of the students. You must be prepared to participate and if necessary suggest changes that would make them work better. There is no point in going to tutorials week after week and muttering afterwards 'That was a waste of time'. Most tutors will be only too happy to have you suggest topics and new approaches which will make the sessions more enjoyable for both them and you.

PRACTICAL LABORATORY SESSIONS

'... to train students in making deductions from experimental data and to foster critical awareness.'

Staff and students alike rank this objective first for laboratory sessions.

Do laboratory sessions have more to offer? Undoubtedly. They develop practical skills, allow you to see how theory ties in with practice and provide training in problem solving and report writing. Some topics are simply most appropriately learnt in an experimental setting. At times you will be collaborating in teams to tackle more complex problems than those that any one person could tackle alone in the available time. The acquisition of these team working skills will be valuable for you throughout your professional medical career.

However, in my experience the amount of time spent on practicals is decreasing. This is for a variety of reasons, but one is that many schools simply do not have sufficient laboratory space and equipment to accommodate 200+ students. Other reasons are the removal of repetitive practicals of little educational value, the replacement of 'wet' practicals by computer-based simulations, and a questioning of the value of some long-established practicals within a medical course as opposed to an honours course in science.

The detail of what you can expect to get from the laboratory sessions and what is expected of you in carrying them out and writing up reports varies from specialty to specialty. But be the specialty biochemistry, physiology, pharmacology or some other, the exact requirement will be carefully explained to you. You will almost certainly be provided with handouts or workbooks describing the practical in advance. *You must read these so that you fully understand what the practical is about **before** you arrive.*

While the detail related to practical work differs between specialties, there is also general commonality. You can identify five basic levels of complexity of practical work, which apply across most specialties (Box 14.2).

Box 14.2 Levels of complexity of practical work
Level 0 — Materials/methods provided to reach pre-determined answer
Level 1 — Materials/methods given but have to work towards answer
Level 2 — Aims and materials given but have to find own method
Level 3 — Aims only given. Have to choose materials and find method
Level 4 — Have to define problem and then design required experiment

Level 0 and level 1 clearly require less scientific thinking than the higher levels. However, they may be useful for training in a particular skill, such as how to use a piece of apparatus. The 'demonstration' is frequently at level 0 but may be useful for reinforcing material learnt in lectures.

Level 2 and level 3 are tightly or less tightly structured exercises which require planning and scientific thought. There is frequently more than one way to solve a problem and in level 3 practicals you can choose the method and appropriate apparatus. A (slightly light-hearted) example of a level 3 practical is 'How do you find the height of a block of flats using up to three of the following pieces of apparatus: a barometer, a stopwatch, string, a metre rule, a protractor and a £5 note?'. There are many possible solutions. Try and think of some.

Level 4 practicals best reflect real-life scientific and medical problems. They may require the work of a whole team, as they tend to involve not only the most interesting problems but also the most complex. They are the sort of problem often tackled in project work extending over more than one practical session.

Within the new courses being developed, you are likely to be moving progressively to higher level practicals in order to develop scientific and problem-solving skills. The advice in the 'Good writing' section of this guide will help you in writing them up. As well as 'wet' laboratory experiments, you will also meet 'dry' practicals. These are simulations, using a computer program to model data. For instance, in pharmacology a computer can model how the level of a drug changes in the blood when a patient develops liver failure or renal failure, which stops the body from breaking down the drug and excreting it normally. The problems computer simulations raise are often extremely challenging. As well as being fun to use and learn from, these programs are of real use. As an example, they are used routinely to adjust some antibiotic and other drug regimens in hospital patients to prevent drug toxicity.

ANATOMY

One rather special area of laboratory work is that in anatomy, which differs slightly from the conventional laboratory classes outlined above. Anatomy covers areas such as gross anatomy, histology and dissection. Much of the dissection will have been prepared in advance (*prosections*) but in some schools you may carry out some dissection in groups under supervision. This helps you to develop manual skill and fix in your mind the inter-relationships of structures such as muscles, nerves, arteries and veins. This is knowledge for which you will be grateful when you are a house officer having to take blood from the femoral vein in the middle of the night ('Now is the vein lateral or medial to the femoral artery that I can feel here?') or tackle your first appendix (supervised).

Anatomy is a subject which students frequently find difficult to learn. *Try to learn it as a visual subject, not as tabulated data.* That is, draw and learn simple line diagrams of muscles, their attachments, nerve and blood supplies and adjacent structures. That way, remembering one simple picture allows you to recall many pieces of related information. Recalling a diagram, stored in a notebook, also passes the time while waiting for, or travelling on, buses. Try working with two or three friends using *learn–teach–taught* circular learning. For example, student A spends an hour drawing and learning simple line diagrams of the upper limb muscles and their relationships. He teaches these to student B in the next few days. The following week he is taught the material by student C, who has been taught it by student D. Meanwhile student B draws and learns diagrams of trunk muscles and student C studies the brachial plexus etc., each cross-teaching and being cross-taught by the others. The efficiency lies in the reinforcement of learning and in having to teach the topic to someone else. This itself is an excellent method of learning.

15

Information technology and informatics: how they can help you

Information technology and informatics are servants, not masters (Fig. 15.1). If you have never used a computer and words such as 'information technology' and 'network' mean little or nothing to you, don't worry. You won't be alone. If you are already, in the jargon, 'computer literate', don't worry either – you will have the chance to improve and expand your skills during your time at medical school.

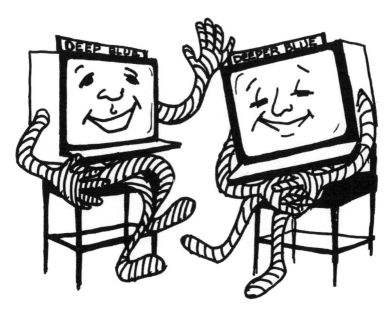

Fig. 15.1   'It's the psychology of the consultation I find so fascinating.'

Common reasons for a lack of basic information technology (IT) skills are lack of opportunity and lack of interest in computers. Provision for developing basic IT skills varies greatly across secondary education in the UK and EU in general, and is even more variable for students from some (but not all) non-EU countries. Mature students may have undergone secondary education when computers were a rarity in schools, and have had little exposure to them. Many students are not particularly interested in computers for their own sake. None of this matters. What does matter is that you understand that a computer is a tool to use to get a result you need. This can be a typed text, a graph to bring together some data, a medical reference from Australia or a set of blood results to help you manage an ill patient. You will need no programing skills during your medical course, and no more than a very general idea of what is going on inside the computer case.

It is likely that early on in the course you will be shown how to use a computer and some common software packages. There are several types of package with which you will rapidly become familiar: word processors, spreadsheets, databases, statistical packages and graphics packages.

Word processors

Used for typing documents. You can delete, insert or move around blocks of text and easily correct your mistakes. Word processors will also check your text for spelling errors. Very useful for the averidj mortal. Is it necessary to be a touch-typist? Well, no it isn't but obviously if you can type 35–45 words/minute you will have an advantage over those able to type at only 10–15 words/minute. If you are unable to type, the University Computing Service will almost certainly have a teaching program that you can purchase for a nominal amount, or have one available over the network. Alternatively, if you want to learn before you arrive at university, a number of commercial programs are available (e.g. *Mavis Beacon Teaches Typing*). Developing this skill will be worthwhile for your undergraduate and early postgraduate career. Voice-operated word processing packages are now beginning to appear, so whether it will be a necessary lifelong skill is in doubt.

Spreadsheets

These are used for storing numerical data from studies and experiments. They allow calculations on data to be performed easily and automatically. Many will also turn the data into a graph for you, to help you appreciate what is happening. An example of their use is to simulate what happens to the blood sugar of a diabetic when you give him/her a meal and various amounts of insulin.

Databases

These are a sort of computerized card index, with the advantage that the computer can be made to do most of the work for you. For instance, if you stored summaries of drug actions on a database you could ask the computer to sort out all those drugs that could not be used in pregnancy, or were useful in asthma.

Statistical packages

For fans and phobics of mathematics alike, these packages take the labour out of statistical calculations. You might use a package, for instance, to help answer a question such as 'Do the female members of your year of the course have a smaller lung capacity than the male members when corrected for body weight and height?'. I don't know the answer.

Graphics packages

These help you to turn your data easily and quickly into different types of graph, such as pie charts and bar charts. They can take the pain out of data presentation.

Computer-based learning (CBL)

The above are all *applications* packages; that is, they allow you to do something quite general, such as word processing any text that you choose or turning any data into graphs. You will also be introduced to computer-based learning packages, which are rather different. They are basically learning aids and range from ones which pose scientific problems or help you to improve diagnostic skills or patient management, to ones which act as electronic 'books'. The best of these 'books' are different from ordinary books. They can include sound and vision sequences, and also guidance so that you can choose your path through them and explore areas of interest in depth. After your introduction to applications packages you will have all the computer skills required to handle CBL packages. CBL is also sometimes called computer-aided learning (CAL).

NETWORKS

Many programs and information resources are accessible through the local university computer network. You connect ('log in') to this with a 'user name', given by the computing service, and a private password which you choose yourself. Typically you will then meet a menu, from which you can select further options. For instance, one option might be to go to the library information databases and then choose one to explore. If you chose Medline you would be able to search several million references and abstracts to find information on some specific topic (e.g. treatment of asthma). Another choice might be to go to the computing service Windows interface, where you would find programs you could run and use in all the areas of applications discussed above plus many more. Most of the navigation is of the straightforward 'point-and-click-with-the-mouse' variety. Technical knowledge of computers is not needed in order to use the network.

This local computer network is known as an *intranet*, and can be used to submit project reports, request help and obtain feedback in some institutions. Rarely is this the case in medicine, as few medical teachers are comfortable with computer technology. The network also acts as a gateway to the world through the Internet (as opposed to the Intranet which serves just the local institution) and World Wide Web (WWW). The Internet is growing exponentially and now allows you to search and extract information from many millions of computers throughout the world using devices known as search engines, which keep a continuously updated index of information available. Search engines are transparent to the user. Again, no technical knowledge is required. The easiest thing is for you to ask someone to show you how to get onto the WWW and perform a search. Try, for instance, looking up information on the new drug riluzole, used in the treatment of motor neurone disease, the debilitating illness suffered by the physicist Stephen Hawking. All that is required is to type 'riluzole' in the 'submit search term' box and press 'return'. Within a few seconds the indexes of millions of computers will have been searched for information on riluzole and a list of relevant articles returned.

The WWW also contains a huge amount of medical information in the form of case studies, tutorials, video clips, multimedia textbooks etc. Try for example the following site:

http://www-sci.uci.edu/~martindale/HSGuide.html

This will give you an idea of the thousands of resources available. A word of warning about the WWW. As it gets busy it slows down, so if you are getting information from the USA do so in the morning, before they are up. Browsing the WWW is great fun and can bring some great information. It can also be overwhelming, addictive and a great waste of time, so distinguish between work and play when using the Web and don't confuse the two.

One of the most common uses of networks is for the transmission of *e-mail* (electronic mail), which allows you to rapidly contact others, whether in Leeds or Otago. The method is straightforward and either it will be explained to you or an explanatory leaflet will be available from the University Computing Service. Your younger tutors (and some of the older ones) will use e-mail. If your tutors do not suggest it, it is worth asking them if you can submit queries to them using e-mail as this can be a great time-saver and aid the planning of tutorials.

INFORMATICS

As well as learning about the mechanics of IT you will learn about the much broader topic of medical informatics. While there is no precise universally accepted definition of medical informatics, the following has been suggested: 'Medical informatics is concerned with assembling, correlating and making effective use of information and decision-making in healthcare delivery'. Put like that it sounds pretty arid, but it isn't really.

Computers have made it easy for us to access vast amounts of relevant information, exchange it with colleagues and plan effective patient management. Systems are now being put into place so that we can use the theoretical benefits of these systems. Inevitably, solutions bring further problems and one of the major areas of concern to those working in health informatics is that of the confidentiality of information. If you were ill in hospital, who would you allow to have unrestricted access to your information? A doctor needing your latest blood results? The dietician providing food supplements? The administration costing your treatment? The hospital porters querying whether you needed an escort to the X-ray department? Distant economist looking at the health economics of your condition? Would you yourself want access to all your information? This and many other issues are currently being debated.

While medical informatics is being taught in some form in most medical schools in some cases it is a separate course, in some tied in with IT and in some with another course such as medical statistics or evidence-based medicine. It will become increasingly important in health care and is one of the several new disciplines already putting pressure on attempts to reduce curriculum overload by demanding its place in medical courses as part of the core content.

TO BUY OR NOT TO BUY?

In theory your medical school/university will provide computing facilities for your needs, but there are still arguments for having your own computer. First, medical schools are all cash-poor so facilities are often limited. This is one of the few areas in medical education which is unlikely to change over the next decade. Second, human nature being what it is, projects get left until the last minute so that several hundred students end up trying to print out their reports 2 hours before the last ('Yes, I really do mean no further extensions.') deadline and the system cannot cope. Third, the main university network may be accessible only from computer clusters on campus or in halls of residence. Not the most convenient arrangement if you want to work late at night or surrounded by books, draft documents, cups of coffee and the cat.

If you are not an IT aficionado you must take advice before you buy. If you are an expert, still read through this section in case there is something you have not considered. Currently (1998), a new computer will cost you £800–1600, plus another £150–200 for a colour-capable ink-jet printer. £1600 will get you a machine from the high end of the range: more speed and memory than you will ever need, full multimedia capability, massive hard disk storage, fax/modem, quality software. A joy, a tool and a toy. (And an insurance headache: university flats and residences are 'high risk' – you may find both a £500 excess and a £1000 limit on any claim.) The lower end of the range will give you a computer which is perfectly adequate for producing your reports, essays and analyses and which 3 years earlier would have had a performance considered to be 'at the top of the range'. Computer technology progresses fast. Second-hand machines have little value and new machines once purchased, drop in value faster than holly after Christmas. So, decide what performance you want and don't chase the technology.

Your University Computing Service (UCS) can give good support. They frequently buy from one major supplier whom they know provides quality, value products, and students can also purchase these machines through the UCS at very good prices. The UCS can advise what software packages it supports and what is installed on the local network. While converting files between major word processing packages is generally not difficult, it does save hassle and the occasional problem if you are using the same product on your home PC and on the network. The major software companies offer students some excellent integrated software packages (e.g. Microsoft Office) at a fraction of the normal retail cost; enquire from the UCS. Other major suppliers offer a recent version, but not the latest, very cheaply (e.g. Corel WordPerfect). This is not altruism – they know that if you start using a product you tend to stick with it for years and at some stage will upgrade, earning them bucks.

A word of warning about upgrades. A few years ago a word processor provided everything you needed to produce quality reports: it required 4 MB of RAM and a few megabytes of hard disk space. It suited the PC it was on. Updating to the latest version may give you a product which promises you the capability of producing the *Encyclopaedia Britannica* with embedded sound and graphics. The small print also says it will require 32–64 MB of RAM, 100 MB of hard disk space and the fastest processor on the market. If it does not have these it will run slower than the old version, if at all. So be careful, think before you upgrade software and ask yourself what the new version will offer that you actually need and will your machine be able to run it. Never be afraid to seek advice.

There is a perennial argument between a group of PC users and devotees of Apple Macintosh (Mac) computers about the relative merits of their machines. It is an exceedingly tedious argument. They are exceedingly tedious people. If your university is PC-based, buy a PC. If it is Mac-based, buy a Mac. If it is both, then go with the flow worldwide and buy a PC. Until recently relationships between Microsoft and Apple were akin to those between the Montagues and the Capulets, but financial strains at Apple have recast Microsoft as both suitor and provider of a dowry. Whether the outcome will be any happier than that for Romeo and Juliet remains to be seen, but many see Bill Gates as an improbable Romeo.

If you do decide you need a computer, here are six suggestions for you to consider:

1. Apply to a medical school which supplies each student with a portable PC. (Newcastle is the only medical school I know of which is piloting this, but things may change.)

2. Suggest to your parents that the 3-year-old home PC is hopelessly out of date, they need an upgrade and consequently you will look after the old machine for them. This was my daughter's approach.

3. Share a flat with a good and generous friend who owns a PC and preferably has different working hours from you.

4. Suggest it as an 18th birthday present, getting-into-university present from doting relatives, etc.

5. Pay £500 or less for a machine no more than one generation old in the processor stakes, with its original software (e.g. if Pentium was current then 486 would be acceptable). Make sure it has a provenance and an identity number – many advertised in the press and around universities are stolen. (Beware of nearly new 'bargains' for the same reason.)

6. Take out a bank overdraft. I do not advise this unless after several months at medical school you really cannot manage without your own computer.

Remember that the medical school *must* provide reasonable facilities for you to be able to carry out your programme of study. If there are difficulties with computing facilities and you do not have your own, then discuss this with your tutor.

16

Early clinical contact

Increasingly clinical contact begins during the first year of the course, frequently within the first few weeks. This can be daunting as your knowledge is limited, the professional doctor–patient relationship is new to you and many feel uncomfortable touching another individual who is a stranger, even with permission. These concerns will all be familiar and understood by those you are working with. Many of your tutors will remember their own first encounters: the dryness of the mouth, the shakiness of the hand, the feeling of the mind going blank as you grope for a sensible question to ask next. It all soon passes.

Early clinical contact is likely to be in situations such as a general practice or other community health setting, a casualty department, an outpatient clinic or with a particular patient group which has offered to help. One of the things that comes out of early clinical contact is the start of a growing knowledge base, centred around the clinical cases you see, but there is much more. When observing, think about things such as the following.

How does the clinician interact with the patient? Does he/she greet the patient, identify himself/herself, explain who you are and why you are there? Is the patient offered 'the option' of your being present? Does the clinician alter his/her approach and explanations according to the age, gender, ethnicity and educational attainment level of the patient? If so, are the changes appropriate? If you hear medical terms that you do not understand during explanations, then how likely is it that the patient will understand them? What does the purpose of the consultation seem to be?

Traditionally it is assumed that doctors are always trying to find out what is wrong with the patient. You will find that in many consultations there is no firm diagnosis and what is being negotiated is a plan of management which is acceptable to both patient and doctor (Fig. 16.1). Do the objectives of a consultation in general practice and one in a hospital outpatient clinic differ?

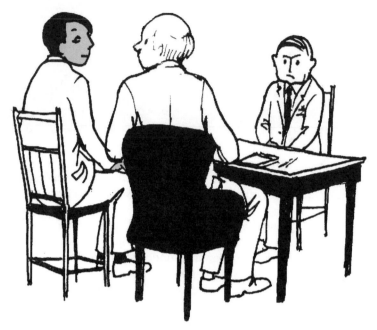

Fig. 16.1 a 'No, doctoring is symptom–diagnosis–tablet. That's all Jones wants.'

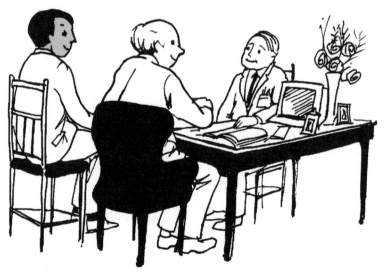

Fig. 16.1 b '...but how have you been feeling in yourself, Mr Jones?'

Think about how you would want to be treated as a patient, and find out whether your views are the same as those of your medical and non-medical friends, and relatives in their forties or seventies. For instance, at a very simple level would you want your GP to greet you by your first name or by your formal title, such as Ms Jekyll? Is the former presumptuous, without your permission, or is the latter inappropriately formal and austere for today's social climate? Is there a right or wrong answer to this?

Think about your own prejudices. We all have them. As you meet a series of patients, what is your initial reaction to them? Depending on your background and experience, it is likely that you will find it easier to empathize with some than with others. How do you feel about those who by their behaviour 'brought the disease on themselves' and are now demanding that you sort it out? Do you find it difficult to relate to a certain racial, cultural or social group, such as New Age travellers? If so, how do you ensure that your feelings do not affect the treatment you give them and, more likely, the time you spend listening to them and explaining things to them? Basically you need an awareness that you do have prejudices, and by being aware of them you avoid adverse consequences for patient care.

How does the doctor relate to other staff and vice versa? What roles do other members of the team have? How do the staff and doctor react to you – do they make you feel welcome or a nuisance?

Early *limited* clinical examination is practised within the peer group in some medical schools, relying on student volunteers. Many dislike the thought of being touched by strangers. If you do, especially consider volunteering. This will give you an appreciation of the feelings of your patients and, being on the receiving end, you will know which of your colleagues made you feel at ease and comfortable and which made you feel embarrassed or vulnerable. At no medical school should you be forced to act as a surrogate patient against your will, but you will be expected to learn the required clinical skills by examining others and these may include fellow students if this is the method of teaching used. If you are unwilling to be examined at all, e.g. having power, tone and reflexes in your upper limb tested, it may be important to discuss with your tutor why you have such strong inhibitions as it could affect your ability to examine others fully. Initial shyness is not uncommon and there may be cultural, religious or ethnic reasons, all of which will be dealt with sympathetically, but you may need to discuss them.

The move to early clinical contact is one of the great advantages of modern courses and is the part of the course that students generally enjoy most. Not surprising really as, for most, clinical work is why you came to study medicine.

17

The clinical firm

While *Tomorrow's Doctors* advocates a move away from strictly discipline-based teaching, you are likely to find that much of your hospital experience is based around a clinical firm. This will probably be the way in which your clinical learning opportunities are organized even if you are not to be instructed in the complexities of the firm's discipline. Thus, on a surgical firm you should not learn the details of laparoscopic surgery but the patient undergoing laparoscopic surgery will be the focus for teaching opportunities. For instance, you might consider issues such as informed consent, the different roles of those working in the ward team and the concerns that individuals have on coming into hospital for procedures which we consider 'routine'.

The structure of the clinical firm was well established and essentially uniform until recently. The consultant had ultimate responsibility for the care of the patient and was supported by junior staff. Supporting staff were senior registrar (occasionally), registrar or senior house officer (SHO) and house officer(s) (HOs). House officers were frequently in their first year after qualification, known as the preregistration year, and were then known as PRHOs. Two or three consultants, usually in different specialties, shared some of the junior staff and had their patients concentrated on one or two wards. 'Outliers', a consultant's patients off their main wards, were looked after by the same junior staff – a chore if there were many outliers. This system is easy for you as a student. You get to know and be known by the consultant and junior staff. It is easy to identify them as being responsible for your teaching and to find out what is going on and who has been admitted. This is the traditional structure, which you will know of from TV and films and discussions with those already qualified. Incidentally, the term 'junior staff' is a misnomer for qualified professionals who could be over 30 years of age with 8 or more years of experience. It is a long-standing public relations and professional negotiating 'own goal' by the medical profession.

Many hospitals have now moved away from this structure to structures such as a 'ward-based' system, mainly because of a reduction in junior doctors' working hours. There has also been a change in junior doctors' training, with a more structured and shorter training programme before inclusion on a specialist register from which they can apply for consultant posts. The more structured programme has less service commitment and a greater educational component. Registrars and senior registrars in training posts have been amalgamated into a specialist registrar grade (SpR).

Ward-based systems vary but typically the HO and SHO look after all the patients on a given ward, whichever consultant the patients are under. They do not look after outliers, and may well not know of their existence. This can make life for students difficult if they are consultant-based and expected to know all their patients, even if not on their main ward. The specialist registrar may remain consultant-based and be your best source of information. If outliers tend to go to one of only a couple of wards, a member of the student firm needs to have the responsibility of checking those each morning for newcomers. If you are ward-based yourself, rather than consultant-based, you are likely to be required to clerk all patients on the ward whichever consultant they are under. In this structure, arranging the satisfactory discussion of cases and teaching may well be exceedingly difficult. If the system does not seem to work, clarify by discussion with your medical school. Personal uncorroborated observation is that consultants working with the above type of ward-based system become prematurely grey.

An alternative type of ward-based system does not have the above disadvantages. Here, a consultant and his junior staff have responsibility for all patients on a given ward. Once the ward is full, patients go to other consultants depending on which wards have empty space. The advantages claimed are that multiprofessional team working is easier, consultants' workloads are more evenly distributed and junior staff do not waste time walking round the hospital from ward to ward. There are potential disadvantages. Some continuity of care may be lost as it may not be possible to hand back readmitted patients to their previous consultant if that consultant's beds are full.

18

Working on the wards

'There should be no teaching without a patient for the text and the best teaching is taught by the patient himself.'

(William Osler, 1903)

The asthmatic so short of breath she can no longer speak. The smoker with angina, now admitted with a heart attack, fingers still nervously rolling a final tab. The young teacher with diabetes, unconscious due to low blood sugar. The man with too-long-ignored rectal bleeding, now coming in for the too-late resection of his colon cancer. The patients who you will see on the wards will mostly be at this end of the disease spectrum. Often they will have an underlying condition which you have met before when it was less severe. Inpatients generally fall into two main categories. First, people who have been admitted acutely with conditions requiring hospital care, such as the first three above. Second, those admitted for a procedure or investigation which is most conveniently carried out as an inpatient. This group includes 'list' admissions for surgical procedures, such as the last example above.

You will be expected to clerk these patients and follow their care while they are in hospital. A few of the patients admitted acutely may be too ill or distressed to be clerked by a student but most are not – if in doubt, ask one of the doctors or a senior nurse. You will also of course always seek the agreement of the patient concerned. To gain most from this opportunity you need to talk to the patients every day to follow their progress, follow them while they go for any investigations and accompany them to the operating theatre if they go for surgery. Clerking them gives you a chance to learn about their condition and follow its management, from acute presentation to resolution. Equally important, talking to them every day allows you to gain their confidence and an understanding of what the condition means for their everyday life and what are their concerns and worries.

You should be given a timetable on joining the firm and an introductory talk about what is expected of you and what you can expect. Teaching sessions and their type (teaching ward round, bedside case presentation, side-room tutorial) will be identified, as will sessions which you are expected to attend. These will include things such as X-ray meetings, at which cases relevant to your firm are discussed, and general clinical meetings suitable for a wide range of doctors and students. In some units these tend to discuss the rare and exotic, so do not be too worried if you fail to understand everything being discussed. The timetable will also cover outpatient sessions you may attend (usually on a rota), business ward rounds and 'takes'. Ward rounds are either business rounds or teaching rounds. On the first you can expect to learn by observation about patient care and management but there is likely to be only limited teaching, especially in a very busy unit. Depending on the case mix, your stage in the course and the clinicians involved, the value of business rounds varies from very considerable to limited. On teaching rounds you can expect discussions to be much more focused to your needs, and opportunities for such rounds should not be missed – not least because the responsible student often has to present the case, so your absence is evident. Combined teaching and business rounds are often more successful in the later stages of your clinical studies.

All the medical staff on your firm have a responsibility for student teaching except perhaps for the house officer, who is considered to be undergoing a year of supervised training before full registration as a doctor. In practice, house officers often provide much informal teaching and advice and students perceive them as being more approachable than senior staff. Indeed, they may have known the house officers while they too were students. Others involved in patient care will often be willing to explain what they are doing and what they have to offer. These include physiotherapists, occupational therapists and speech therapists as well as various specialty nurses (cardiac rehabilitation, respiratory and diabetic care, stoma care, etc.). Understanding the breadth of their contribution will make your life a lot easier when you qualify, so take opportunities to see them at work. An informal individual approach is most likely to be successful and fruitful.

'Takes', when your firm is responsible for the day's emergency admissions, allow you to see cases at their most acute and often most dramatic and memorable. They often give you the chance to practise newly developed skills such as taking blood or inserting cannulae and putting up drips. Most emergency cases are admitted outside the hours of 9–5. You are likely to be resident (on a rota) within the hospital for some of these take periods. You can expect suitable accommodation and a 'bleep' so that you can be called to cases when they arrive and be involved in their diagnosis and early management. This is an extremely important part of your medical education: your social life takes second place!

When you start on your firm you should be given, as well as the routine information discussed above, information on how you will be assessed and whether there will be a chance part-way through the firm to discuss your progress with a tutor. This discussion helps to plan the clinical experience you need in the later part of your attachment to the firm.

As a firm of students, much responsibility for organizing learning opportunities may lie with you. Expect to elect a chief clerk, who will record all admissions which are the responsibility of the student firm and allocate them promptly among the students. Do not be too reluctant to take on this task – a moment's reflection and you will realize its potential advantages. Organize a method of exchanging information about interesting cases and physical signs so that learning opportunities are not missed and identify areas in which you feel you need teaching. Ask teachers to help cover these topics. Give some warning, 24 hours if possible, and try to identify a couple of appropriate cases to hinge the teaching around. Record topics that you have covered and those you still need to cover using your learning objectives for the course or logbook if you have one. If you are not pro-active in planning your teaching you may find that on disorganized firms the teaching becomes limited in scope and repetitive. Try to work co-operatively. If you have clerked a patient who is going for an investigation take a second student along – but first present the case to that student as you would on a ward round or teaching round. Observe each other examining patients, using check-lists to help provide feedback. Sample check-lists for respiratory, cardiovascular and abdominal examination are given in Boxes 18.1, 18.2 and 18.3. They may be photocopied and enlarged. You will see that there is no similar check-list for neurological examination or sections of it. After a few weeks on the ward, work with a colleague to make one up.

The main thing on clinical firms is to make the most of your opportunities. See as many cases as you can and read up just a little on each case. Your future skill as a diagnostician will largely depend on your case experience. And remember, when clerking and examining patients do not assume that just because they have been seen by someone senior there is nothing new or different to find. In the week of writing this chapter, two new students with 1 week of clinical experience identified by careful examination a patch of pneumonia and pleurisy in an elderly lady on my ward. She had been diagnosed by qualified staff as having only musculoskeletal chest-wall pain a few hours before. What you do can make a difference.

Box 18.1 Examination of the respiratory system

Use this list for peer practice with a colleague. The following should be covered. The list is *not* comprehensive, but designed to form a basis for discussion and improvement. Mark as Yes, No or Not Applicable and add any comments required.

GENERAL

Introduced self to patient	Y	N	
Due regard to patient comfort/modesty	Y	N	
Self: appearance/dress appropriate	Y	N	
Self: manner considerate/friendly	Y	N	

INSPECTION

Chest adequately exposed	Y	N	
Position: directly in front/behind patient	Y	N	
Chest shape/symmetry checked	Y	N	
Scars noted	Y	N	
Respiratory pattern/rate noted	Y	N	
Peripheries inspected	Y	N	
Checked for cyanosis/anaemia	Y	N	
Peak expiratory flow rate checked	Y	N	
Sputum pot checked	Y	N	N/A

PALPATION

Trachea/apex beat checked	Y	N	
Expansion UL/LL front/back checked	Y	N	
Vocal fremitus checked	Y	N	
Lymphadenopathy checked	Y	N	
Breasts checked	Y	N	N/A
Permission to check breasts requested	Y	N	N/A

PERCUSSION

Bases checked	Y	N	
Apices checked (front/back)	Y	N	
Axillary regions checked	Y	N	
'Hands-on-head' position used	Y	N	

Box 18.1   Examination of the respiratory system (contd)

AUSCULTATION

Methodical (front/back/axillae)	Y	N	
Normal/abnormal breath sounds noted	Y	N	
Normal/abnormal voice sounds noted	Y	N	
Abnormal added sounds noted	Y	N	
Patient aided to dress	Y	N	N/A
Patient thanked	Y	N	
Differential diagnosis made	Y	N	
Required further tests formulated	Y	N	
Overall technique fluid/methodical	Y	N	
Overall patient approach satisfactory	Y	N	
Further attempt required/problems identified	Y	N	

Overall comment (Give POSITIVE feedback first!):

Name: Date:

(May be copied complete and enlarged for individual/firm use.)

Box 18.2   Examination of the cardiovascular system

Use this list for peer practice with a colleague. The following should be covered. The list is *not* comprehensive, but designed to form a basis for discussion and improvement. Mark as Yes, No or Not Applicable and add any comments required.

GENERAL

Introduced self to patient	Y	N
Due regard to patient comfort/modesty	Y	N
Self: appearance/dress appropriate	Y	N
Self: manner considerate/friendly	Y	N

INSPECTION

Chest adequately exposed	Y	N
Appearance noted (pale, anxious, sweating, scars)	Y	N
Respiratory pattern/rate noted	Y	N
Visible pulsation noted	Y	N
Peripheries inspected	Y	N
Checked for cyanosis/anaemia	Y	N
JVP: patient position correct	Y	N
JVP: height and waveform checked	Y	N

Box 18.2 Examination of the cardiovascular system (contd)

PALPATION

BP checked (technique, Korotkoff)	Y	N
Radial pulse (rate, rhythm)	Y	N
Central pulse (oharacter)	Y	N
Trachea/apex beat checked	Y	N
Thrills (precordium/carotids) checked	Y	N
Parasternal heave	Y	N
Hepatomegaly/hepato-jugular reflux	Y	N
Peripheral pulses/radio-femoral delay	Y	N
Oedema (sacral/ankle)	Y	N

PERCUSSION

Bases checked	Y	N
Cardiac dullness checked (rarely relevant)	Y	N

AUSCULTATION

Heart sounds (base/apex)	Y	N	
Heart sounds (intensity)	Y	N	
Added sounds noted	Y	N	
Murmurs noted	Y	N	
Murmurs timed from arterial pulse	Y	N	
Position to check for aortic incompetence correct	Y	N	
Position to check for mitral stenosis correct	Y	N	
Bell/diaphragm usage correct	Y	N	
Carotids/femorals (if required) checked for bruits	Y	N	
Bases checked for crepitations	Y	N	
Patient aided to dress	Y	N	N/A
Patient thanked	Y	N	
Differential diagnosis made	Y	N	
Required further tests formulated	Y	N	
Overall technique fluid/methodical	Y	N	
Overall patient approach satisfactory	Y	N	
Further attempt required/problems identified	Y	N	

Overall comment (Give POSITIVE feedback first!):

Name: Date:

(May be copied complete and enlarged for individual/firm use.)

Box 18.3   Examination of the abdominal system

Use this list for peer practice with a colleague. The following should be covered. The list is *not* comprehensive, but designed to form a basis for discussion and improvement. Mark as Yes, No or Not Applicable and add any comments required.

GENERAL

Introduced self to patient	Y	N
Due regard to patient comfort/modesty	Y	N
Self: appearance/dress appropriate	Y	N
Self: manner considerate/friendly	Y	N

INSPECTION

Abdomen adequately exposed	Y	N
General appearance (wasting/bloating)	Y	N
Visible peristalsis/scars/pulsation noted	Y	N
Peripheries inspected	Y	N
Checked for anaemia	Y	N
Cutaneous signs noted	Y	N
Oropharynx and dentition examined	Y	N
Flanks and loins compared	Y	N

PALPATION

Enquired for tender areas	Y	N
Superficial and deep palpation	Y	N
Liver and gall-bladder examined	Y	N
Spleen examined (including right lateral position)	Y	N
Both kidneys palpated	Y	N
Other masses examined	Y	N
Good palpation technique	Y	N
Lymphadenopathy checked	Y	N
Groins/hernial orifices checked	Y	N
Permission to check above requested	Y	N
Anorectal examination considered	Y	N
Permission to perform PR requested	Y	N

PERCUSSION

Ascites	Y	N
LKKS (liver, kidneys, spleen) and other masses as appropriate	Y	N
Abnormal pattern of resonance	Y	N

Box 18.3 Examination of the abdominal system (contd)

AUSCULTATION

Bowel sounds (character/absence)	Y	N	
Bruits noted	Y	N	
Patient aided to dress	Y	N	N/A
Patient thanked	Y	N	
Differential diagnosis made	Y	N	
Required further tests formulated	Y	N	
Overall technique fluid/methodical	Y	N	
Overall patient approach satisfactory	Y	N	
Further attempt required/problems identified	Y	N	

Overall comment (Give POSITIVE feedback first!):

Name: Date:

(May be copied complete and enlarged for individual/firm use.)

19

Learning in outpatient clinics

Outpatient clinics offer both opportunities and difficulties to the student. Some advantages are listed in Box 19.1.

Box 19.1   Pros of outpatient clinics

Different disease mix
Different disease severity
See natural history of disease
See an emphasis on management
Learn focused history taking
See consultant-junior staff interface
Learn about written communication

Many of the cases you see are rarely seen as inpatients. For instance, in gastroenterology clinics you see patients with dyspepsia (indigestion) and minor bowel problems, such as irritable bowel syndrome, constipation and diarrhoea. Along with these you will see many patients whose disease is currently not of a severity to require inpatient care. In gastroenterology clinics these include patients with chronic liver disease, inflammatory bowel disease, biliary tract disease and pancreatic disease. Many of these will *never* require inpatient care, and they provide a welcome balancing perspective of the varied natural history of many conditions.

Working in clinics lets you talk to patients about their perspective of disease, which may be quite different from that of the doctor. Take an example. Studies show that doctors focus on the physical limitations of chronic diseases such as multiple sclerosis, whereas patients place far less emphasis on these as affecting their quality of life and are more concerned about factors such as their overall mental health and vitality. Interferon beta is a treatment for multiple sclerosis which can be shown to decrease the rate of development of new lesions. It is very expensive and it is a natural, although illogical, human reaction to believe that patients should be particularly grateful for the provision of an expensive treatment. However, the treatment causes reactions at the injection site, flu-like symptoms, nausea, muscle pain, fever, depression and malaise. These decrease the patient's quality of life in an immediate way while treatment does not even guarantee the lack of disease progression in the future. Talking to a patient who has suffered these side-effects you can appreciate why patients become 'non-compliers' with the treatment we prescribe. Much of outpatient consultation is not about diagnosis. It is about the negotiation of a management plan between doctor and patient, when each of the two has a different agenda for what he/she wants to achieve. Think about the agenda of each as you listen to the consultation.

You will learn a different style of history taking and examination in outpatient clinics compared with that on the ward, an approach much more akin to that you will meet in general practice. History and examination are targeted on the system involved, with less attention being paid to other systems which are unlikely to be relevant. You may well meet a requirement for a focused history or examination during your clinical exams, in either short cases or an OSCE (objective structured clinical examination, described in a later section). Focused techniques are well worth practising, both for these and for your later professional work. Time constraints do not allow a 'complete' history and examination of all patients at every visit, nor would the yield of useful information be sufficient to make this worthwhile.

Take the opportunity to read patients' referral letters. These will usually be from a GP; some will be from a hospital-based doctor. Ask yourself a few questions. Are they legible? Is it clear why the patient has been referred and what the GP wants? Some may be requesting a diagnosis and management, others may want to manage the patient themselves after a diagnosis. Some may just be wanting a professional colleague to reassure a concerned patient. Does the letter contain the details you need? For instance, since patients rarely know the names of the tablets they are on this is very useful information – as is information about any concerns that the patient may have but may not be prepared to divulge to a strange doctor. As an example, a young man with diarrhoea and weight loss may have an underlying fear of HIV infection following travel in Africa, and this type of information is helpful in a consultation.

Look at the letters from hospital to GP. When were they sent relative to the date of the clinic? Was the delay likely to cause problems for the GP? (I worked in a hospital with an 8-week delay, and was reduced to faxing handwritten notes or phoning in the case of serious problems.) Was the information given to the GP what he/she would need, and did it answer the questions asked in the referral letter? Did it say what the hospital was going to do by way of things such as ongoing follow-up or joint management? Did the letter say what the patient and/or relatives had been told?

You will also see how the consultant interacts with the junior staff in clinics, what cases he/she allocates to them and discusses with them, and the sort of queries that they bring to him/her.

Outpatient clinics can teach you a lot about different aspects of patient care, as well as being a source of 'interesting physical signs', but in practice students often find that the sessions are unrewarding. Some of the disadvantages of clinics are shown in Box 19.2.

Box 19.2   Cons of outpatient clinics

Time limited
Teaching limited
Random sample
Repetitive
Purpose poorly defined

Clinics are busy and there is rarely any concession in the schedule to the presence of students. This limits direct teaching to a few minutes per patient at the most, and if clinicians get behind they may stop teaching until they catch up. Patients often appear in random order, which can be confusing for the student. The patient with irritable bowel is followed by the one with fibrosing alveolitis, by the one with Crohn's, by the one with primary biliary cirrhosis. Very confusing. At the end of the 40 minutes you are left wondering whether Crohn's disease is the same as colitis and what the consultant meant when he/she told you the patient had primary biliary cirrhosis but told the patient that his/her liver was not cirrhotic and in fact it was functioning fine. Alternatively, you spend an afternoon in which everyone seems to have irritable bowel syndrome or non-ulcer dyspepsia, there have been no 'physical signs' and you wonder whether your time would not have been better spent in the library or playing a game of tennis. If you find you are in either of these two situations, do three things. First, for any new condition you have met, read it up after the clinic and make a few notes covering such standards as aetiology, presentation, main features, management and prognosis. The notes should be the equivalent of only half to one side of A4 paper. Second, read the section above about the advantages of outpatient clinics, and consider these factors in the consultations. Third, consider discussing a reduction in the time you spend in the clinic. It may be better to attend for only half the clinic. This can relieve pressure on the clinic doctor, who can then crack on for the first half of the clinic and allot some teaching time to the second half. Before suggesting this compromise, and explaining the thinking behind it to the consultants, sound out their likely reaction from the junior staff – some consultants may consider the proposal a personal affront!

The above represents the situation with most outpatient clinics. A few of you may be fortunate enough to work in a hospital with planned teaching clinics. The number of patients is reduced to allow plenty of time for the students to clerk, present and be taught on the patient. The patients have previously agreed to being clerked by students and often there is a clinical theme running through the cases which helps learning. An example of such a theme is a clinic with eight to ten patients, each of whom has shortness of breath on exertion for different reasons. While becoming more common, such clinics are still the exception. They have advantages in terms of structured teaching about conditions, presentation and management. However, even if you do enjoy their advantages take care that you do not overlook the more indirect opportunities for learning in routine clinics, discussed above.

20

Working in primary care

Work in primary care forms an important part of your course, whether or not you intend to work there, because that is where the bulk of medical care takes place.

As well as working with a GP you are likely to see the scope of the work of the practice nurse, district nurse, health visitor, receptionist and others. Work in primary care is, of course, not limited to work related to general practice but involves work in other areas as well. Some examples are discussed in the sample paediatric course outlined in Chapter 5 on the core curriculum. All medical courses provide an opportunity to work in at least one general practice but the number and total time involved varies from course to course. A common pattern involves two general practice attachments with different patient populations – perhaps an inner city practice and a town/rural practice. Additionally, time will be spent with the university department of general practice preparing you for your attachments. Currently, the total time on your course spent working in general practice is likely to be 4–12 weeks. Reasons why this may increase are discussed towards the end of this chapter.

What might you expect from your time in general practice? Patterns will vary, but the following is an example. The attachment takes place during the second half of the course, after a period of clinical training within a hospital. Initially, work in the department of general practice covers discussion of the basic consultation, video recording of practice sessions with tutor feedback, giving information to patients (for instance on diabetes mellitus) and difficult consultations (for instance, counselling after a miscarriage). These are all small group sessions and, after some initial apprehension over being recorded, are enjoyed by most students. This initial period provides orientation as to the nature of general practice and a first insight into a different form of practice from that you have seen in hospital (Figs. 20.1 and 20.2).

Two 10-day general practice attachments follow. Practices are not required to take students, so those that do are welcoming and friendly. In turn they expect you to bring enthusiasm, open-mindedness to a different approach to health care and a polite, caring approach to the patients you see. Many of these will have been looked after by the practice for decades gone and will be for decades to come, so you will not be popular if you treat them roughly or inconsiderately! You will be expected both to observe and participate. Within the practice you work mainly with one GP, but also with the partners, and spend half-day sessions observing the work of others involved in the care of patients. Initially you sit in as an observer during consultations, but soon you will see and examine patients on your own and then present them, discuss them and plan their management with the GP. The history and examination are focused on the system concerned, rather than following the totally encompassing approach often taught in hospital. You

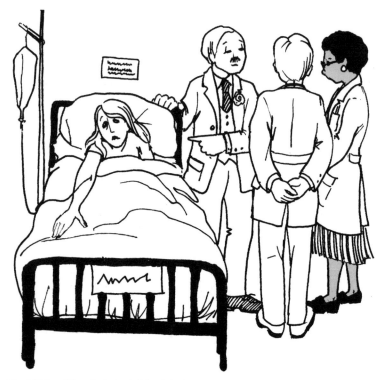

Fig. 20.1 'Alison is just a brittle diabetic.'

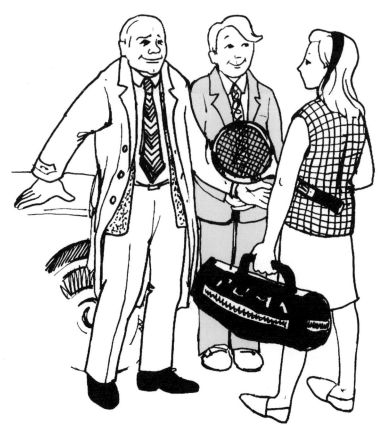

Fig. 20.2 '...but you don't let the diabetes stop you doing things, Alison, do you?'

will have direct observation and feedback on your clinical techniques, and these will improve rapidly as tuition is on a one-to-one basis. One of your GP attachments is likely to be residential so that 'out of hours' calls can be attended. The practice may cover all of its evening and night calls or a patient 'drop-in centre' may be used for some calls, especially in the early evening (before, say, 10 p.m.). These centres, which are staffed by GPs, deal with patients from a group of practices and are useful for patients with transport who do not need a house call.

The patients you see will have been asked for their permission for you to sit in on or undertake the consultation, and occasionally they will refuse permission. Do not take this as a personal slight. It may be that they feel uncomfortable discussing some particular intimate problem with someone they do not know present. It may be that they would never wish a third party to be present, even if they were consulting about a common cold. This is their absolute right and no comment on you personally.

In hospital it is difficult to gain experience in many procedures and assessments because there are so many other students around, but often general practice provides you with these opportunities. Examples include passing a vaginal speculum; breast, pelvic and other intimate examinations; applying dressings; developmental assessment of children; and assessment of things such as how sick a child is or whether the child is seriously dehydrated.

Hospital is often also a very foreign environment to patients and relatives, and the way they normally interact is easier to see when they are in the surgery or you are on a home visit. For instance, how confident is the 4-year-old? Does the child cling to mum's skirt while you talk to her, or go and play with the toys in the corner of the surgery? Do mum and child seem relaxed together or is mum showing signs of unusual stress through her words and body language? Observation is a key skill, enabling you to gain information from the patient's and relatives' demeanour, appearance, manner and body language, whether in the surgery or the home (Fig. 20.3). Home visits will show you the variety of ways in which people live. Malnutrition and squalor exist in houses sporting satellite dishes and with a car parked outside. Family violence, children abused and on the at-risk register and those with psychotic mental illness exist right across the social spectrum, as indeed do children in loving, stable, caring families, whether adequately off or poor. Perspective is different in general practice. In hospital we tend to view illness as being the focus for the patient. We feel annoyed when someone stops taking the treatment we prescribed for their moderate but symptomless hypertension. In general practice you understand that the priority was cash for a day out with the kids or some school games kit, not for more tablets which anyway make them feel dizzy. A different focus.

As well as seeing many patients in the surgery and on day and night calls, you will be asked to see and write up a patient in depth. This will give you the chance to explore how the disease affects not only the patient but the whole family. It will be someone with chronic disease or disability, or a very elderly patient. You will see how his or her care is shared between practice and hospital, where appropriate, and discuss the adequacy of letters linking care between the two.

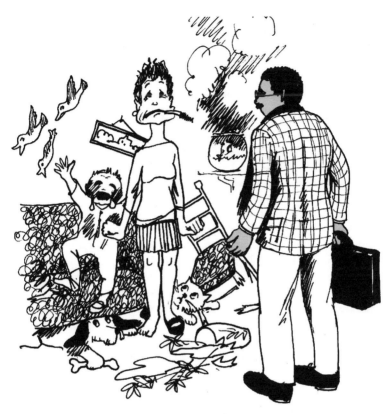

Fig. 20.3 'Tense, TENSE, *TENSE!* What makes you say *that?'*

Work will also be with other members of the healthcare team. These will include the district nurse, health visitor and practice nurse. Their work includes things such as providing general advice on health, inoculations, dressings, and helping patients in the home (for instance with washing and hygiene). With the health visitor you will visit families with babies and young children from 10-days-old to school age, and learn what problems they face, including developmental checks, feeding problems and those on the at-risk register. With the receptionist you will learn phone-answering protocols and how cases are classified as urgent, routine or requiring discussion with the doctor. And you will learn how they all work together to provide efficient care.

Students are often greatly changed by their experience in general practice. They tend to come away with a new respect for the service, and often also a realization that they had been unaware of how much clinical care is undertaken in general practice and by comparison how little GPs refer patients to hospital.

I mentioned at the start of this chapter that the pattern of GP attachments could be changing. This is due to the changing focus in the medical course with earlier clinical contact, increasing numbers of students and decreasing numbers of hospital beds. The proposal is that much of the early stage of clinical aspects of training should be in general practice rather than in hospital. After all, the basic skills of history taking and examination can be taught in either and the population of patients in general practice is huge. Students would be more easily taught in small groups, of perhaps four, which would allow observed practice and feedback. Note that this is not about more teaching of the specialty of 'general practice' (although many would argue for this), but about the teaching of early clinical skills. My personal view is that such changes are feasible but would not be cheap to implement and monitor. GPs' routine work would be severely disrupted and whereas current attachments may slow the work it remains manageable. There is a big difference between teaching one student and teaching four – bigger in many ways than a change from four to twelve. All this means not that the change should not take place but that it needs to be adequately piloted and funded so that it remains enjoyable and fruitful for both provider and recipient in the long term. GPs in the Hunter Valley, New South Wales, have made a major contribution to the community-based medical course at Newcastle (NSW) for many years, so stable arrangements can be developed. Even if basic clinical instruction is moved to general practice, the types of attachment currently undertaken are likely to continue to be an important and enjoyable part of the course. Make the most of them.

21

Learning communication skills

If you look up the word 'communication' in a dictionary, you find it defined along the lines of 'act of imparting (especially news); information given'. It is something you do every day: talking face-to-face or by phone, or sending messages by letter, fax or e-mail. Why then do medical schools feel they need to teach it explicitly?

Until recently they didn't. Communication skills were learnt, as was much of clinical medicine, by observation of your clinical tutors and by osmosis. These methods depended heavily on your good fortune (or otherwise) in your allotment of tutors and the situations they met and dealt with when you were with them. The main reason for the explicit teaching of communication skills is that the types of skill you need in medicine are different from those that you need in much of everyday life. The situations that you meet will probably be outside your experience prior to medical school. This will be true not only for those who come direct from school but also for mature students, except perhaps those who have already worked in the healthcare professions. A secondary reason is that perhaps because of the way 'communication' is so often defined in a dictionary it is thought of as a process in which transmission, rather than reception, dominates. In clinical medicine the reverse is most often true. The third reason is intensely practical. The majority of the growing number of complaints against doctors relate to issues of communication, both oral and written, rather than to issues of poor professional standards. Good communication can avoid many of these complaints and the consequent stress for patient, relatives and, not least, yourself as a doctor.

There is no exact definition of 'communication skills' common to medical schools, but a dichotomy exists between those schools which largely equate communication skills with consultation skills and those which perhaps take a broader view and start at a more general level. A dichotomy also exists between those who believe that communication skills can be taught and those who believe that they are largely intrinsic to individual personality, and are modified by experience and growing maturity. Be assured that many studies in the literature do show that communication skills can be developed through good teaching courses.

The schools which equate communication skills with consultation skills tend to concentrate on clinical situations, using discussion and role play to tackle difficult areas. Examples of areas you might cover include the clinical history, giving information, breaking bad news, dealing with the disturbed or aggressive patient, talking to children, cross-cultural communication and taking a sexual history. In a session on 'giving information' to a patient, you might cover the setting (private room/open ward?), seating arrangement and use of appropriate vocabulary. 'Appropriate vocabulary' means avoiding jargon and ambiguity and matching the vocabulary to a person's educational background. Other aspects tackled might cover providing space for the person to ask questions, to clarify information and just to talk/reflect; making a contract for a further meeting if required; and a discussion of where you both want to go next in managing the consequences of the information. You will cover much more, but the above indicates how 'giving information' might extend beyond the content of the information given.

Sessions may be on the lines of 'paper cases' used as a basis for dicussion, or may use actors/fellow students and video recording to simulate real situations. While you may find the thought of being recorded while tackling a difficult situation daunting, in my experience the tutors on such courses are invariably positive and your fellow students act as supporters not aggressive critics. Sessions also look at aspects of communication such as that between members of the care team; written communications, such as discharge letters and the keeping of case notes; and telephone and fax transmission, including issues related to confidentiality. With the previous preclinical/clinical divide, 'consultation skills' were principally taught from around the third year of the course when clinical work largely started. With the move to earlier clinical contact, consultation skills teaching has increasingly moved to earlier in the course. The instructors most frequently have a background in medicine, and may be GPs who also take students on attachment. This form of 'consultation skills' training is largely that which I have described in the previous chapter on work in general practice and in hospitals.

Schools which look at communication skills in a broader context than that of the clinical consultation have been able to start teaching communication skills from the first year of the course even when, as in the past, that year contained little clinical contact. Often the early years of these courses have a greater emphasis on generic communication skills and personal effectiveness skills than on communication skills particular to the medical context. By generic skills I mean communication skills that would be of value in almost any field of study or occupation. Examples include the skills of establishing rapport, active listening, presentation, team working and providing feedback. Personal effectiveness skills assist other communication skills. They include skills such as time management, managing stress, oral and written presentation, tolerating ambiguity in decision making and effective study skills. Simple exercises in studying listening skills might involve looking at the use of body language to encourage or discourage someone to talk, or making enquiries of sales staff in stores to see what methods they use to encourage you to purchase goods. These courses are often organized by psychologists or behavioural scientists, which adds a different overall flavour to the course.

Which approach is best? Neither. Some of you will learn more from one approach, some from the other, and some would benefit equally from either. Most will be learnt by using your course as a framework on which to build over your undergraduate and post-graduate career. A side-benefit for many students is the finding that, although they are not in the top half of the class in terms of knowledge of factual material, they can contribute at least as well as the academic high-fliers in many areas of communication. In truth, you are more likely to be well thought of by your patients if your communication skills are good and your knowledge adequate than if your knowledge is state-of-the-art but you are considered not to have empathy with those to whom you are talking/listening. *Note, however, that clinical knowledge must always be at least adequate! Empathy is no excuse for ignorance.*

22

The clinical skills learning centre

There is one development in the UK in the field of medical education which is even more recent than *Tomorrow's Doctors*. This is the establishment of a clinical skills learning centre (CSLC) in the majority of medical schools. Here we will look in a good deal of detail at how these can work, as they can provide you with a new, versatile and powerful way of learning much material in a fashion different from both the traditional apprenticeship model and working in the library.

As CSLCs are still developing what follows is based largely on my own experience in setting up a very successful and popular CSLC in Leeds but also draws on many fruitful conversations with others, across five continents. Even the title, CSLC, is not settled. One school's CSLC is another's clinical skills laboratory (CSL) or clinical skills centre (CSC).

CSLC RESOURCES

Let's look first at the types of resources available in a CSLC and examples of how they can be used to form your own learning package or in set workshops. Resources typically include manikins, videotapes and laserdisks, computer-aided learning (CAL) programs and links to Internet resources and reference sources (such as Medline). Apart from general space, many CSLCs also have a communication skills suite.

'Manikins' are models on which you can practise procedures away from the patient. (As opposed to 'mannequins', who are generally employed by designers to model clothes and costumes). You are possibly familiar with the Resusci-Anne manikin used for teaching basic life support, but a wide range is available. Some examples of skills that can be taught on manikins are: basic life support, retinal examination, venous cannulation, arterial blood gas sampling, lumbar puncture, urethral catheterization, pelvic examination, breast examination and prostatic/rectal examination. Videotapes cover topics such as how to take a history or examine a particular body system (e.g. the respiratory system or abdomen) at elementary and more advanced levels. Others cover specific techniques (e.g. putting in a central line or performing a lumbar puncture) or topics (e.g. interpreting the ECG, the management of meningitis or parents' views on how they were told of the diagnosis of meningitis in their child). A CSLC might have a range of 50–100 or more videotapes.

Laserdisks typically contain 11 000 to over 30 000 clinical images, and some contain sound or video sequences as well. A laserdisk is basically a very large slide collection with consistent high quality and no jamming, scratched slides or 'someone seems to have borrowed those we wanted' slides.

CAL programs have improved tremendously over the last few years, in part following the development of CD-ROM, with large storage capacity and rapid access. The best CAL programs are truly interactive. Examples are simulations, case management programs, tutorials and text. Consider a simulation concerning diabetes. This might start off with a diabetic whose diabetes is out of control so that the patient is dehydrated, has a very high blood sugar and is acidotic. You have to plan how much insulin to give and at what rate, how you are going to replace the fluid deficit, plus anything else you think necessary. Depending on your choices the patient stabilizes, improves or gets worse and then you have to take further action on these results until the patient is 'cured' (or 'killed' if things go badly wrong). As you can imagine, practice on such simulations is not only far safer than using a real patient but also far less stressful.

Case management problems are also interactive. Typically, you take a history, perform an 'examination' and make a tentative diagnosis. Using a figure on the screen and point-and-click-with-the-mouse cursor, you examine the patient. Examples of the type of examination you can perform are that you can ask to hear heart sounds, watch a video of the patient's gait or ask for the blood pressure or the results of examination of the abdomen. Having made the diagnosis you can order the normal range of tests and interpret them yourself or ask for a report. As all tests are costed, wastage is discouraged. If you get stuck you can 'phone' for expert advice but usually you reach a diagnosis. At this stage there is a comparison with the expert approach to the diagnosis and a discussion of management, likely outcome and prognosis. These problems are powerful aids to learning.

CAL tutorials provide short teaching sessions on specific topics like interpreting heart and lung sounds or X-rays, or managing asthma, and often tie in with case management problems. A large number of standard medical textbooks have been transcribed on to CD-ROM. Often the publishers have made no concessions to the change of medium, and reading page after page of text from a monitor screen is a tiring and not very rewarding process. You may well prefer the paper-based textbook. Other publishers have made good use of the new medium and have used devices like animated diagrams to aid understanding. Look at what is available and judge for yourself whether to use them or the paper-based versions.

Resources on the Internet are growing exponentially. Now, from a single Internet site you can access many tens of thousands of different items of teaching material, and these will become an increasingly used resource over the next few years. Limitations at the moment include speed of data transfer and congestion which slows traffic on the Internet.

A CSLC will also have teaching space and areas for talking to and examining peers, simulated patients or real patients. It will in addition have a communication skills learning suite, and this is discussed later.

USING THE CSLC AS A RESOURCE FOR DIRECTED SELF-LEARNING

Only limited by your imagination. An example. You have been talking with a man who has heart failure and who was booked for an echocardiogram. Despite the introductory course talk that you had been given on history and examination, you felt you couldn't fit his story together. When you examined him you were unsure what you were supposed to be looking for and the meaning of what you found. The chest X-ray looked pretty fuzzy compared with the few others you had seen, and you had been told 'You should look at his ECG'. The SHO had agreed to discuss the case with you, but she seemed awfully busy and had now disappeared. There was no one else around to ask. A not uncommon situation.

You and two others go to the CSLC to ask for help. The teaching assistant there discusses your priorities. It is early in your clinical career. Learning about history and examination comes first. Then possibly a little bit about chest X-rays and the management of heart failure. ECGs can come later, although the CSLC has some videos and CAL programs on ECGs. The CSLC also has a CD-ROM on 'Transoesophageal echocardiography' with seductively beautiful colour video sequences, but that is postgraduate material for budding cardiologists – not for you. A learning resources pack to meet your needs is put together (Box 22.1).

Box 22.1   Learning resources pack: cardiac examination/heart failure

Video: 'The cardiovascular system (CVS) history'
Video: 'The cardiovascular system (CVS) examination'
'Clinical examination' text, to clarify any points
Check-list on CVS examination (prepared by CSLC)
Peer practice at CVS examination, using check-list
CVS examination observed by teaching assistant (20 minutes)
CD-ROM: 'Physical signs': sections on cardiology and heart failure
CD-ROM: 'Heart and lung sounds': sections on normal sounds and those in heart failure
Review patient on ward
Notes on how to look at chest X-rays (CXRs), supplied by CSLC
CD-ROM tutorial on CXRs and examples of CXRs
Standard student textbook: section on management of heart failure
CD-ROM tutorial on heart failure
Interactive case study relating to heart failure

You choose from these resources those you want to use to meet the learning objectives you have identified. After 5 hours' work you feel more confident about cardiovascular examination and identifying heart failure. You also have some idea as to how it should be managed. This learning has taken place by your own efforts, with just a little guidance to help identify appropriate resources.

This is one example but similar learning packs can quickly be put together to meet many of your learning needs, and you will soon get to know what the CSLC has to offer. *Note that the work of the CSLC is to support and complement your face-to-face clinical learning, and is not to replace it.*

USING THE CSLC FOR SET WORKSHOPS

Some skills are needed by all students and are best learnt initially in a CSLC rather than on a ward. For example, it is unacceptable to attempt to insert a urinary catheter or put in an intravenous line unless you are familiar with the equipment, the method, the approach to the patient and the sterile technique required. Workshops in the CSLC provide an environment which is safe for you and not time-constrained. No patient is put at risk and you can practise a procedure until you are confident. Discussions about technique, alternatives and complications, which are difficult or inappropriate around a patient, can take place over a manikin. The manikins which are available are not perfect, but provide reasonable simulations. While set workshops vary between CSLCs, common examples are intravenous cannulation, basic life support, retinal fundoscopy, urethral catheterization, pelvic examination, breast examination and presenting a case history.

Each workshop has a number of set objectives, and combines learning resources and teaching methods to achieve them. Take a workshop on retinal fundoscopy. Examination of the back of the eye using an ophthalmoscope enables the clinician to identify changes in the retina and the blood vessels running across it. Changes may suggest that a disease, such as diabetes or hypertension, is present. An ophthalmoscope is a hand-held device with a beam of light and lenses which enables you to look directly through the pupil and see the retina clearly. The technique is difficult and requires practice, a methodological approach and an understanding of what you are looking at. The main objectives of this workshop are that you, the student, should be sufficiently confident afterwards to use an ophthalmoscope on patients during routine examination and also should be able to pick up signs of hypertension and diabetes. You should be able to describe what you see and have some idea if 'something doesn't look right' so you can ask for a more experienced opinion. An outline of a workshop for six to eight students, lasting about 60–75 minutes, is given in Box 22.2.

Box 22.2   Outline of a workshop on retinal fundoscopy

Video on how to examine the retina
Four-stage silent run-through
Examination of fundus by fellow students
Practise on manikins
Review of fundal pictures on laserdisk
Practise on patients (wards/clinics/GP)
(Other resources)

The workshop would be facilitated by a tutor, who could be a doctor, a teaching assistant or a suitably trained more senior student. The video shows students how to hold and use an ophthalmoscope and describe what they see, and gives examples of the normal, hypertensive and diabetic fundus. A 'four-stage silent run-through' is a standard teaching technique, in four stages as the name suggests. First, the tutor examines a subject's fundus without explaining the procedure, to give an overview of the whole. Second, he/she repeats the examination, saying what is being done and looked for. Next, a student describes what the tutor is doing during the examination, but just slightly ahead of what is being done. Fourth, a student (not necessarily the same one) does the examination and describes what he/she is doing stage by stage. The repeated reinforcement makes this a very powerful and versatile teaching method.

Students then examine each other's eyes in a darkened room or with artificially dilated pupils to make it easier. They learn practical details, like why you use your right eye to examine the patient's right eye, and why long hair is best tied back. (To avoid intimate face-to-face contact and stop loose hair flapping in the patient's face respectively.) The tutor is available for discussion. Practice follows using manikins, which are model heads in which 35-mm slides of various retinal conditions can be placed at the back of the 'eye' to mimic pathology. The laserdisk is used to review, discuss and describe the normal, diabetic and hypertensive fundus. Students have read up on the changes over the previous week, so have substantial background knowledge already. Clinical practice takes place after the workshop to reinforce what has been covered.

Open access to the CSLC means students can come back to review material if they feel the need or to look at further related material on video or CD-ROM. This covers topics such as how to detect corneal ulceration or remove a superficial foreign body. (I recall caustic comments from a then girlfriend when, as a fourth-year medical student, I did not know how to evert an eyelid to remove a chunk of a fly that had flown into her eye and lodged there. It proved to be a closing chapter in our relationship.)

The above shows how learning resources and teaching methods can be combined to provide a valuable learning session. Students find this more interesting and worthwhile than either a lecture on 'Looking at the retina' or immediate exposure to a diabetic clinic, where they do not know what they are looking for or how to use the equipment, and are rushed owing to the clinic being busy. Clinical time is valuable and patients are the most valuable teaching resource. Workshops make sure that you can make best use of that time and resource. *Again, note that workshops are to complement clinical work and not to replace it.*

TEACHING SKILLS IN AN ATTITUDINAL AND KNOWLEDGE-BASED FRAMEWORK

In Leeds, I developed an approach to teaching skills which involved an appropriate framework of knowledge and attitude, rather than skills in isolation. Other units may prefer a more technical, skills-based approach, teaching the attitudinal base separately – perhaps as part of a communication skills course.

If you look at the list of examples of set workshops you will see that some are nearly totally skills-based, with a knowledge element but little attitudinal element – for example, the basic life support workshop. Others have a greater attitudinal element. In the workshop on intravenous cannulation, attitudinal issues such as prior explanation to the patient and whether or not to use local anaesthetic to limit patient discomfort are discussed. Inserting an intravenous cannula will be an everyday event to you but may be a unique and important life-event for the patient, and this is also considered. In other workshops it is important to discuss attitudes, and the skills component is relatively minor. In the workshops on breast examination and pelvic examination, the technical aspects of the video and the manikin practice take only a minority of workshop time. The majority of time is spent in discussion about attitude. How do you approach someone to request an intimate examination such as breast, pelvic or rectal? What are the patient's likely concerns and how can you limit his/her discomfort and embarrassment (and yours)? What are your feelings towards the individual, as a patient and as a person? Do they differ from those of your colleagues? How do feelings vary according to gender and cultural and religious background in the examiner and the examined? All these types of issue can be discussed more easily around a manikin than around a bed. If discussions take place within a group whom you know and trust many anxieties can be dealt with before you have to perform your first intimate examination, under guidance, on the ward.

COMMUNICATION SKILLS TEACHING SUITE

A CSLC will contain various tutorial rooms and IT facilities but it will also contain one very important room, the communication skills teaching room. This is traditionally a room divided by a one-way window. Efforts at taking a history or handling a case presentation, as you would on a ward round, or at breaking bad news to a 'relative' can then be watched by a large group without their presence being obvious and disturbing the process. Now, the one-way window has often been replaced by an audiovisual link so that efforts can be not only observed, but also recorded and used for later feedback sessions with those involved. A study of recordings results very rapidly in improved presentation and consultation skills. It often becomes apparent early on how much time we spend talking when we think we have been listening to the patient!

MULTIMODAL APPROACH TO CLINICAL SKILLS TEACHING

The above examples show how teaching can be integrated in two ways in the CSLC. First, resources such as manikins, videotapes and CAL are integrated. Second, the knowledge, skills and attitudes components can be integrated. In the more complex workshops, the range of resources is increased and other, wider, skills and attitudes can be developed. Take the following example of a workshop centred around the topic of 'meningitis'. Objectives are set (Box 22.3) and resources are supplied (Box 22.4).

Box 22.3   Objectives of a workshop on meningitis

At the end of the workshop the students should:

1. be aware of the clinical presentation of various forms of meningitis
2. understand how to perform a lumbar puncture
3. understand CSF (cerebrospinal fluid) changes involved
4. be able to plan appropriate therapy
5. be aware of modern developments in, and limitations to, prevention and therapy
6. understand the anxieties of parents and relatives
7. have improved their ability to use Medline on the network
8. have improved their communication, group working, presentation and teaching skills
9. have achieved other objectives, as determined by the student or group.

Note the last objective.

Here you see that a wide range of skills is developed, including those related to time management, presentation, planning and group working. The need to share tasks has also to be understood as not all the objectives can be met by any single individual in the

---

Box 22.4   Resources for a workshop on meningitis

Resources provided include the following. The numbers in parentheses refer to the objective(s) (in Box 22.3) to which the resources are mainly linked.

1. Manikin for lumbar puncture (2)
2. Video of (a) expert clinical discussant on meningococcal meningitis and (b) interviews with relatives of patients with meningitis, and subsequent studio panel discussion (5, 6, 8)
3. Summarized histories of 15 cases of meningitis or suspected meningitis, with CSF (cerebrospinal fluid) results and treatment regimes (1, 3, 4)
4. 'Mock' case histories; colour prints of meningitic CSF in counting chamber; and 'CSF' samples, for sugar estimations for match and diagnostic exercise (1, 3, 4, 7)
5. Literature on prevention by vaccination and public health measures, related to forms of bacterial meningitis (5)
6. Medical textbooks and access to Medline via network (7)
7. Frames on meningitis from National Slide Bank laserdisk (1, 3)
8. Actress (or role play) for parent of child in mock case (6, 8)
9. OHP and whiteboard facilities (8)
10. Some refreshments half-way through session (1–9!)

---

time available, even in a half-day workshop. Priorities must be set and the group must decide which objectives they must all meet (e.g. practising a lumbar puncture on the manikin, experience of breaking news to a relative) and which can be tackled by some and reported to others (e.g. literature on prevention of meningitis, modern trends in therapy). Skills such as time management and presentation skills are known as 'transferable skills'. That is, they are skills which are not specific to medicine but which will be of use to you throughout your professional medical career or any other profession you may eventually choose.

This use of the CSLC to provide multimodal, broad-ranging workshops depends on the culture of the student body. This culture is increasingly to wish to pursue directed self-learning, rather than be given a didactic course of study with little variation to suit students' particular needs and interests.

23 Assessment

This chapter has three main purposes. First, to look at the reasons for assessment. Second, to look briefly at some of the educational vocabulary associated with assessment. Third, to discuss a form of assessment – group project assessment – that you may meet during your course which has not been covered elsewhere. More familiar forms of assessment are discussed in the chapters on MCQs, clinical exams and writing an essay.

REASONS FOR ASSESSMENT

It may seem strange to have a section on 'why we assess'. Many academics believe the answer is obvious: if we do not assess, our students will learn nothing. Not only do I disagree with this belief, but I know that we assess for many much more complex reasons. These include internal factors and also satisfying external elements who have a legitimate interest in the standard of medical education and include the Higher Education Funding Council, the General Medical Council, UK and EU statutes, trust hospitals and the public.

External bodies which are keepers of the public purse must be satisfied that they are getting value for money, and those bodies with statutory responsibility for the standard of medical education must be satisfied that appropriate standards are being met. This is one reason for the external examiner system within universities. In this system an academic from another institution becomes one of the examiners, and can look at standards more objectively than the internal examiners and from a different viewpoint. It is also necessary to satisfy those who are going to employ our graduates – initially mainly NHS trusts – and the public, who will receive their care, that standards are satisfactorily maintained. UK medical degrees are recognized by many other countries whose hospitals have similar interests in quality to our own.

Internal factors justifying the assessment of students include the more obvious of ensuring that students are reaching the standard required to progress through the course (summative assessment) and also that our courses are teaching what we intend (course/teaching audit). A further, major reason for assessment is to provide student feedback so that students can improve their knowledge and performance – so-called formative assessment. These types of assessment are considered in more detail below.

EDUCATIONAL VOCABULARY

In medicine there is a lot of jargon, a professional vocabulary that allows you to exchange ideas and concepts efficiently with other professionals. Among educationalists there is jargon too, albeit different, and some has already been discussed earlier in this book. Now is the time to introduce and explain a little more – that which you are likely to meet in your course. The ideas I want to introduce are those of summative and formative assessment and of criterion-based and norm-referenced or peer-referenced assessment. Also, a few further definitions.

Summative and formative assessment
Summative assessment is judgemental, to see how well you have performed on your course. Although you may see the results, as with A level grades, this assessment is basically designed to meet the needs of some other individual, body or institution. This may be your teacher, course organizer or prospective university. If you have done well, you will not be told where you excelled. If you have done badly, you will not learn whether the deficit was global or patchy. Summative assessment frequently has a gatekeeper function to control the flow of students through a course.

The primary purpose of *formative* assessment is to help you, as a student, to develop. You are given feedback and discussion as to where your strengths and weaknesses lie. You may well be given an overall mark but this is not the most important aspect of the assessment. A growing number of assessments in both clinical work and non-clinical work are of this type.

Formative and summative assessment are not mutually exclusive. However, effective formative assessment often requires you to reveal and discuss 'weaknesses' and 'lack of experience' so that you can work out with a tutor ways in which you can be helped. This is beyond the courage of most of us if we are simultaneously being summatively assessed.

Norm-referenced or peer-referenced assessment

You will doubtless be familiar with this form of assessment. Your results are ranked along with those of your peers and your position is judged relative to them. The crude scores may be adjusted in some way, for instance to bring them into line with those of last year's students, but your overall ranking relative to your peers will not change. There may be a cut-off point, such that the top 5% get a gold star and the bottom 10% get the opportunity to resit. The decision is taken not on absolute criteria but on relative criteria. Applicants to medical school are effectively ranked and selected. Many applicants who are not selected would doubtless pass the course and make good doctors. While scores may be manipulated so that they have a 'normal distribution' (a bell-shaped curve), this is not necessarily the case for the term norm-referenced assessment to apply.

Criterion-referenced assessment

In this form of assessment, your performance is judged as far as possible against an absolute standard. If you meet the criterion you pass, if not you fail. At the funfair if you are over 150 cm tall you may ride on the big dipper, if not you can't. You pass your driving test if your standard of driving meets the pre-set requirements. Whether you pass is not affected by the previous five candidates all hitting the kerb, or by the fact that they all could have applied for membership of the Institute of Advanced Motorists. In clinical terms, criterion-referencing makes a lot of sense. We want to know that those we allow to graduate have the necessary skills to perform tasks to a required level of competence. Employers, the public and, indeed, the graduates themselves require the same reassurance.

Validity and reliability

A test is said to be *valid* if, when interpreted, it measures the characteristic that we intend to be measured. If performance in a clinical examination predicted the level of future diagnostic skill, the assessment would be valid if that is what it had been intended to predict. On the other hand, if it had been intended to predict doctor–patient empathy it might not be valid.

A test is said to be *reliable* if the results, when interpreted, measure in a consistent way. For instance, if a group of teachers use a test instrument to rate a given group of students and all the teachers come up with a similar result, the test instrument is likely to be reliable (but it may nevertheless be inappropriate and therefore invalid).

Validity and reliability are often described in terms of shooting at a target of concentric circles. Valid and reliable shooting will group the shots in the bull's eye, where they are wanted. If all the shots are pulled to the right outer of the target, the shooting is reliable but not valid. If the shots are scattered all over the target, the result is neither valid nor reliable and few conclusions can be drawn.

Note that although we often speak of 'a valid test', this is just shorthand – it is not the tests themselves that are intrinsically valid or reliable, it is the way that the test results are interpreted for a defined purpose. An MCQ (multiple choice question) paper might be valid and reliable when interpreted as a test of factual knowledge, but not as a test of clinical problem-solving skill.

Usability/practicality/manageability

These features of a test indicate whether it is a test which can actually be applied in a given situation. Limiting factors may be related to complexity or cost of administration, time needed for administering the test, the skill of the assessors and the ease of scoring the test. For intance, you might wish each student to be examined on 20 clinical cases to provide a broad spread but considerations such as confining the exam to a single day may mean that each student can be examined on only six cases and judgement has to be made on this more limited sample.

GROUP ASSESSMENT

One of the trends throughout higher education, and not just in medicine, has been a shift towards the assessment of some work on a group basis rather than on an individual basis. This is for two reasons, the first often overemphasized by the cynical. That first reason is the growth in student numbers and the decline in numbers, both relative and absolute, of those available to do the teaching within universities. Whereas before (with classes of 60) it was perhaps feasible for two tutors to double-mark an essay, with classes now running into several hundred this is no longer practical. There is just not the academic time available.

The second reason is more complex. Many 'real-life' tasks are not dealt with by individuals but by groups who work co-operatively and produce one outcome or report. The move to include such group tasks in the curriculum means that it is often difficult to identify absolutely the contribution of one individual and, indeed, it is divisive and disruptive of group activity to do so. The logic of giving a 'team mark' is counterbalanced by the desire of many students that their individual effort be rewarded, and certainly that another student should not freeload on their efforts. Another feature of group tasks is that often all the topics are relevant to all the students in the class, but each topic is tackled by only one group of them. Involving students in the assessment of each other's work, so-called 'peer assessment', means that they all learn from each other's efforts. Using forms of presentation with readily assimilable visual impact helps this intergroup learning. A poster from the Leeds students' HIV project is an example of such a form of presentation (Fig. 23.1). The students produce a wide variety of posters. Using both tutors and students to arrive at a mark allows students to see the tutors' approach to assessment, especially if a structured marking proforma is used.

The methods used to allocate marks are various. There is no 'correct' method. Examples are:

1. Allocate the same mark to all students in the group. For instance, all six members get 55%.

2. Allocate an overall mark to the group and allow its members to divide it between themselves as they feel appropriate. For instance, the total mark is 330 for six students and they may allocate this between themselves, by agreement. There must be guidance as to what should influence the distribution of marks: efforts in research, presentation, ideas etc. There must also be an appeals mechanism for any student who feels unfairly treated.

3. Allocate the same mark to each student in the group and also give them a float, to be divided by negotiation between the group members and then added to the first mark. For example, each student is given 45% and the group is given a float of 30 marks to divide between six of them. This can become interesting if the pass mark is 50%!

4. Divide the project into subsections, and give a mark to the student (or pair of students) responsible for the subsection and an overall group mark for the whole project.

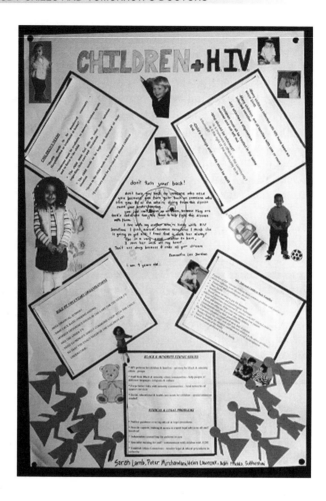

Fig. 23.1 Sample of year one students' HIV project poster. (Original in full colour.)

I will conclude this section with an example of a well thought-out group marking scheme used by the University of Nottingham as part of its microbiology course and coordinated by Tony Short, Senior Lecturer in Physiology. Part of the course has to deal with 22 topics related to antimicrobial chemotherapy and related infectious diseases and pathogens. Each topic is divided into subsections, typically four, and each subsection is tackled by a pair of students. The overall topic is presented using a poster format, with brief oral presentations to peers and members of the academic staff. Examples of topics include: 'Papilloma virus: transmission, epidemiology, role in cervical cancer, treatment'; 'Scabies: the mite, disease, epidemiology and control'; and 'Hepatitis B: virus and pathogenesis of infection, management, carrier state, implications for the medical student'. Marks for accuracy are given for each subsection on a predefined scale of 4–10 ranging from 'grossly misleading' (4), through 'mostly sound, but several omissions or two major errors' (7), to 'well selected, correct material' (10). The same mark goes to both of the students producing each subsection. A second mark is given for 'impact' of the whole poster. 'Impact' is scored from 0–10, a mark of 0–2 being given for each of five components (clarity, layout, colour, interest, lettering legible at 2 m). The marks for accuracy and impact are *multiplied* (an unusual feature) to give an overall mark.

The work of the 180 students involved produces 22 displays, many of which are used subsequently for the teaching of senior undergraduates and postgraduates. The assessment process takes 4 man-hours, and so is practical from the point of view of the department. In addition, the students learn from all the other posters so it is highly efficient for them as well. The standard of presentation of the posters is very high.

Group work and group assessment are features to be welcomed, not feared, in the new medical courses. They offer both variety and experience relevant to your future career in medicine.

24

MCQs

Multiple choice questions (MCQs) are commonly used to test a wide range of knowledge quickly and easily. They can be marked rapidly and objectively, using optical card-readers. They are efficient at testing factual knowledge, and can be adapted to test understanding and some aspects of problem-solving skills.

Books of sample MCQs in most subjects are available in the library. If you use one of these during revision, make sure that you understand the correct answer and how it relates to the topic being considered as a whole. *Do not try to remember hundreds of dissociated facts.* Such a surface learning approach could lead to disaster. Ask individual departments whether they have any sample MCQs, so that you can test yourself to see how your revision is going. Check whether you will be filling in a card to be read by an optical card-reader, and if so make sure you have seen one before the exam (and know whether it is up to you to supply the marker pencil!). A typical card contains columns of boxes numbered to correspond with the parts of each question, and you shade in these boxes depending on your choice of answer so that they can be read and scored automatically by the optical card-reader.

As well as marking each candidate's card the examiners look at the overall performance of the class in each question and identify things such as which questions are highly discriminatory between good and bad candidates and whether there are areas in which teaching needs to be modified. Occasionally, they discover questions which are being incorrectly assessed. Find out how the MCQs are to be marked. Commonly, there is a question followed by five or six statements which you can mark as 'True' or 'False'. In some cases there is a 'Don't know' option (see Box 24.1).

Box 24.1   Example MCQ, seeking factual information

Qu. 27. The following features support a diagnosis of Addison's disease:

1. An eosinophilia of under 1%	T	F	DK
2. A raised level of serum growth hormone	T	F	DK
3. A serum sodium of 125 mM/l	T	F	DK
4. Increased pigmentation of old surgical scars	T	F	DK
5. Symptomatic postural hypotension	T	F	DK

Marking schemes vary. Commonly one mark is given for a correct answer and no marks for 'Don't know'. Marking more than one option will commonly result in zero marks or, if there is negative marking and the examiners are aggressive, a negative mark. For a wrong answer there is either *negative marking*, in which one mark is deducted (e.g. for saying an answer is True when it is False), or there is *neutral marking*, in which no marks are given or deducted. It is your responsibility to find out and understand the marking scheme before you sit the paper.

In neutral marking there is no disadvantage in guessing. In fact, if a *neutral* marking system is being used you *must* attempt all the questions, otherwise you will penalize yourself heavily. For example, in a question with five options of which two are true you will get two marks by marking them all as true (or three by marking them all as wrong), but none if you do not attempt the question. In such neutrally marked papers you may be given only True and False options, with no Don't know category to help you avoid penalizing yourself.

In the case of negative marking, advice varies. Your primary concern is to pass the exam. I would suggest that you *give answers if you know, or think you know, they are correct*. If a guess would be a true random guess, I would suggest that you leave it as 'Don't know'. By random guessing you may gain a few extra marks, but you may also lose a few. The majority of people pass MCQs. The pay-off of random guessing – being ranked a few places higher among the pass candidates – is negligible. The consequence of dropping into the fail category because your random guesses were 'unlucky' – having to resit – is considerable. One student I know set out to beat the system by analyzing old papers and finding that 55% of options were true and 45% false. He reasoned that if he did not know the answer, then he should mark it as true on a 55:45 odds basis. Good logic. He came unstuck, because the options for questions to which he did not know the answer were not distributed in the same ratio. Ultimately, the choice of when and whether to guess is yours. Others' advice to you may differ from mine – it is a topic on which mathematicians publish books discussing 'best' strategy.

In *Gulliver's Travels*, the Big-endians and the Little-endians (in opening eggs) were both passionately convinced that they were right. Similar passions over the relative merits of negative and neutral marking are held in committees, but (although I personally prefer neutral marking) I suspect that whichever is used it makes little difference in practice to who passes and who fails. Supporters of negative marking say that it discourages guessing and that some wrong choices would be dangerous in clinical practice, and so deserve to be penalized by a negative mark. Supporters of neutral marking point out that the random guess element can be corrected by a simple adjustment and that negative marking schemes also are manipulated so that the scores fall between 0% and 100%. They suggest that a small number of candidates are so horrified by the thought of getting a negative mark that they are unable to make a decision and fail to express the true extent of their knowledge: 'the rabbit in headlights' reaction.

The example question given above in Box 24.1 is the most common type, seeking factual information. An example of an MCQ which checks understanding involves students reading a clinical paper and then answering questions such as those in Box 24.2.

Box 24.2   Example MCQ, checking understanding

Qu. 5. The clinical paper you have read:

1. Describes a placebo-controlled study	T	F	DK
2. Describes a single-blind, randomized study	T	F	DK
3. Has a power of 90% (*use the table provided*)	T	F	DK
4. Analyzes data on an intention-to-treat basis	T	F	DK
5. Equates clinical and statistical significance	T	F	DK

Nearly always in MCQ exams, you will have to tackle all the questions. You must of course read the instructions and each question carefully, and note how much time you have. Start at the beginning and work your way through. If there is a question you find confusing then mark it in the margin and come back to it. Watch the time. As discussed above, if there is a negative marking system you are advised not to guess. If there is neutral marking you must attempt everything. I emphasize again that you must make sure you know the marking system before you sit the exam. Questions are now rarely ambiguous, and the time allowed is generally adequate. Thus, even if English is not your first language, you should still be OK. However, if there is a word or phrase you do not understand, then ask one of the invigilators for clarification. The questions asked should largely reflect the content of your core curriculum, and may well be derived from one of the recommended textbooks. The days when MCQs concentrated on the obscure small-print topics have largely disappeared.

25

Exam tradition: long case, short cases, viva

Clinical exams must be passed before you qualify. Generally you will have several clinical exams during the course and 'Finals' exams during the last year. These demonstrate that you are clinically competent to work as a preregistration house officer under supervision and that you have reached a satisfactory standard, for a newly qualifying doctor, in a particular area such as psychiatry, paediatrics or obstetrics and gynaecology. No matter what the level of your theoretical knowledge as demonstrated in written exams, if you are not competent clinically you will fail – although generally you have the opportunity to resit once. A few institutions are proposing greater emphasis on in-course assessment, resulting in selected students not being required to take final clinical exams.

Clinical exams are changing, but the traditional format has been a *long case* and several *short cases*. In a long case you fully clerk (take a history and perform an examination) a patient in the way that you will have done many times during the clinical course, then form a differential diagnosis and a management plan. You are then asked to present the salient features of the case to the examiners, demonstrate abnormal physical signs and discuss the case. In short cases you are asked to perform a specific task under observation and, generally, make a diagnosis. For instance, you may examine the hands of a patient with arthritis and be asked to decide if the arthritis is due to rheumatoid disease, gout or psoriasis. Difficult? Not really. You will be using the skills of examination and pattern recognition that you have developed throughout the clinical course.

Who will assess you? Most likely a consultant from your own or a nearby hospital, but sometimes a visiting consultant or professor who is acting as an external examiner. The external examiner system is used by universities as a quality control mechanism to help maintain standards across universities and courses. The external not only examines candidates in the same way as the local examiners do, but also reports back to the university on the standard and fairness of the exam process. Do not panic if you meet the external. It does not mean that you are a borderline candidate. Externals examine a broad range of candidates, although it is true that in some institutions they are asked to look at cases being considered for grading as a distinction or those about which there is particular concern. I emphasize, however, that the bulk of their work involves the more ordinary candidate, so do not fear the external.

Clinical exams are nerve-racking. Students worry about missing a heart murmur or failing to diagnose a rare neurological syndrome. However, if your approach to the patient is correct and your examination technique is appropriate for your stage of the course you will not be failed for missing a tricky diagnosis. Of course, if you fail to note that the patient has had a mastectomy or has a hemiparesis you could be in difficulty, quite rightly. Before your first clinical exam make sure that you have been observed examining patients under exam conditions and can undertake a long-case history and examination in 10 minutes less than the time allowed. If you cannot, then you need more practice. A spare 10 minutes is required so that you can organize your thoughts and think about possible diagnoses, management options and treatment. Who should observe you? Ideally, a consultant who is likely to be an examiner. Ask for such a session, as a substitute for a formal taught ward session if necessary. If the consultant is unwilling then ask a specialist registrar or SHO.

House staff will nearly all have qualified in the local medical school. They are an invaluable source of information as to the types of short case used. For instance, they may tell you that nearly everyone has short cases covering retinal examination, arthritic hands and examination of the respiratory system. This is useful when preparing for the exam. They will tell you horror stories as well – forget those.

The viva voce exam has several functions and limitations. It is not used by all medical schools for all candidates, but in some it is used as a routine part of finals. The viva voce exam, more commonly known as the *viva*, is an oral exam used to test the candidate's knowledge. (The term 'viva voce' means 'with the living voice'.) Viewed by the examiners as a discussion, it is most commonly viewed by the candidate as an interrogation. This is unfortunate as usually the examiners are only too pleased to upgrade any candidate who shows knowledge, understanding and enthusiasm. To the examiner it is the final, slightly uphill, straight. To the candidate it is Beecher's Brook.

The viva is used most commonly in two circumstances: for the pass/fail candidate and for the pass/distinction candidate. The form of the viva is likely to vary. For the pass/fail candidate the examiners will be looking to see whether the candidate has sufficient knowledge and understanding to proceed to the next stage of the course. They are likely, therefore, to restrict themselves very much to the content of the course or core clinical curriculum. If the viva follows a written exam, rather than a clinical exam, the examiners are likely to take the candidate through areas of the paper in which they were weak to see if they can give them a few extra marks. For example, if you failed to tackle the question on non-parametric analysis or did not do justice to the essay on 'Use of information technology in medicine', then by the time of the viva you must know about these topics and have prepared answers to the expected questions. For the potential distinction candidate the examiners will seek more. They want to know if the candidate shows knowledge, understanding and insight beyond the strict requirements of the course and often whether he/she can show originality of thought and defend his/her position in discussion against opposing views. It often becomes something of a gladiatorial contest (Fig. 25.1).

Medical schools have many traditions and there is a mystique surrounding the conventions regarding vivas at some schools. Sensible schools list viva candidates as being assessed for either

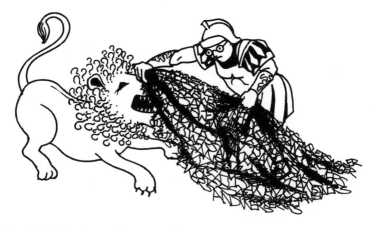

Fig. 25.1 The viva may become a challenging gladiatorial contest.

pass/fail or pass/distinction. Other schools use more subtle differentiation. For instance, two lists – one *inviting* candidates to attend for viva and the other *requiring* candidates to attend. (The first is for pass/distinction vivas, the second for pass/fail vivas.) Such time-honoured subtleties persist, despite the fact that they are incomprehensible to most home students and all overseas students. Candidates should be aware of the level of their viva well in advance so that they can prepare. It is not reasonable for the candidate to walk into a room and be given a viva for pass/distinction when he/she was expecting a pass/fail viva. Or vice versa, and I have met both situations.

Remember, the main reason why people fail clinical exams is simple. *They have not seen and reflected upon enough clinical material.* This is for one of two reasons. They have not done sufficient work overall, in which case they do badly in the written work as well, or they have got the balance of study time between clinical work and theory wrong. This occurs because the responsibility for clinical commitment lies mainly with the student, whereas theory is examined periodically. Clinical practice tends to be neglected in favour of theory. Avoid this mistake, not least because your lifelong skill as a practising physician is founded on your clinical work as a student.

26

The OSCE

While the long case/short case pattern of clinical examination is traditional, a different approach, known as an OSCE, is increasingly being adopted. Because of its growing popularity and its unfamiliarity to many students, I will discuss it in some detail and give an example of an OSCE station.

'OSCE' stands for Objective Structured Clinical Examination. An OSCE consists of *stations* (say 20–30) which you visit in turn, spending the same set time (e.g. 6 minutes) at each. A station consists of a 'task' for you to do, which is assessed in a standard way. Examples of tasks are: to explain to a diabetic how to inject insulin; to examine the respiratory system of a patient; to explain to a man what angina is. An advantage of an OSCE is that we can sample a wider range of skills and attitudes than is normally possible in a traditional exam. Although the performance of a student will vary between one station and the next, by including a large number of stations we can get a fair estimate of the student's ability. The fairness makes the OSCE a popular type of exam with students, especially as the tasks set tend to be clinically relevant. The term 'objective' refers to the fact that each station is marked in a standard way and 'structured' refers to the fact that the exam is set so as to adequately sample in a valid and ordered manner the knowledge, skills and attitudes we wish to assess.

Often the overall question being asked by the examiner is 'Has the student reached a satisfactory standard for progression to the next stage of the course?'. This is called a *criterion-referenced* exam, the criterion being the predetermined level of competence required of the student to pass the exam. Thus in a criterion-referenced exam 100% of the class can pass (only 20% *may* pass, but then you would have to ask questions about the standard of the exam and the teaching!). In contrast some OSCEs are still marked on the basis of norm-referencing or peer-referencing, in which your performance is ranked with that of your peers and a cut-off is made (as is common, for example, at A level). For instance, 70% pass: 30% resit. Criterion-referencing is more logical, but if you are to be peer-referenced then there is probably little you can do about it except discuss the reasons with your tutor. Norm-referencing risks passing students who are not fit to enter the next stage of the course.

Before you take an OSCE there is some information you should try to get. You need to know the number of stations, the time at each station, what type of things will be examined and who will be doing the marking. The time will usually be the same at each station, for example 4 minutes or 6 minutes, because of the way the student body has to flow through the series of stations. It is possible for some more complex stations to take a multiple of the basic time, for example 8 minutes or 12 minutes. There may also be rest stations with no task where you can relax and collect your thoughts. Clinical tasks, such as aspects of history-taking or examination, will be examined but also data interpretation and communication skills may be tested. Marking will be by an observer at some stations but at others the patient may act as marker or the patient and observer both give marks. Even if your task appears to be 'totally clinical', such as listening to a heart, your general approach to the patient and the way you speak to him/her will of course be assessed. A 30-station OSCE can handle only 30 students at a time and so is repeated in several cycles – make sure that you know which cycle of the OSCE to attend and when it starts. We find no evidence that students attending later cycles of the OSCE are at an advantage. We change the data interpretation tasks between cycles, and a few hours' advance knowledge that 'there is a patient with a chest problem' does not help students to examine a chest if they have failed to learn the method over the previous 8 months.

The patients you will meet will be of two main sorts: 'real' patients with a clinical condition, or healthy people simulating a clinical history or clinical signs. Trained simulated patients will provide a history which cannot be distinguished from a real case, and they will reproduce it uniformly from student enquirer to student enquirer. They are less easily fatigued than real patients, and are valued and often very willing volunteers. The Thespian culture is thriving. They can also simulate some physical signs, such as unilateral weakness of a limb, although not others. An enlarged spleen or a heart murmur is outside their repertoire. You may gain an insight into the OSCE by offering to train as a simulated patient early on in the course. Check carefully what will be expected of you. You may feel that having your abdomen palpated by 10 strangers is one thing, but that palpation by 10 students from the year above, who you see on a day-to-day basis, is another.

A great deal more can be learnt from an OSCE if you can get feedback. Feedback is generally of three sorts: immediate individual feedback during the exam, group feedback or individual feedback after the exam. These are considered below.

Some OSCEs provide time for feedback to the candidate at the end of each station, before they move on to the next. The advantages are the immediacy and the fact that the patient can easily contribute. If feedback is given in a constructive, positive manner, even when critical, this method works well. However, if feedback is given poorly and in a confrontational manner the candidate's performance at the next station can suffer.

Group feedback and discussion after the exam can deal with major areas of difficulty met by students, and how their deficiencies can be tackled. The organizers sometimes become aware of areas that they had assumed had been taught during the course, but which had not been covered. It is time-efficient for staff and students to learn from feedback relating to the performance of others as well as their own. If no feedback is offered by a department, suggest using a tutorial session or lecture slot as a group feedback session.

After the exam, one of the organizers may be prepared to discuss your performance with you on an individual basis. It is best to concentrate on identifying areas in which you were strong or weak, and getting suggestions as to how you could improve. For example, you may need to give thought to your communication skills and approach to the patient, or data interpretation may be your problem. Arguing about whether you deserved two marks rather than one for your demonstration of the ankle jerk is not likely to be fruitful. Some departments fear being inundated with 250+ students if they offer this facility. It simply doesn't happen. In practice only those who have to resit, with whom we need to talk anyway, and a few others will enquire. Most students who pass an exam accept the result and move on.

I promised an example of an OSCE station. That described below is a 6-minute station taken from an OSCE set for students on a traditional but changing course, at a time when they had experienced about 8 months of clinical work. It deals with a common and important clinical condition, that of a patient experiencing difficulty in swallowing (*dysphagia*). Given below are the instructions given to the student (Box 26.1) and the information given to the 'patient' (Box 26.2). The 'patient' will have learnt the information in advance, and will use it as the basis for talking about his/her problem. The marking scheme used by

---

Box 26.1   OSCE station on dysphagia: instructions to student

Dysphagia
Take a focused history of dysphagia from this subject, who represents a 60-year-old complaining of things sticking when swallowed.

You will be given marks for taking a relevant history. You will also be given a few marks for telling the examiner, after taking the history, what is likely to be wrong with the patient and for suggesting two relevant investigations that would help you to confirm your proposed diagnosis.

(You can talk freely in front of the 'patient' to the examiner about the diagnosis suggested by the history – the 'patient' is acting.)

Box 26.2   OSCE station on dysphagia: instructions to 'patient'

Dysphagia station
Please offer appropriate information only in response to questioning.

You are a 60-year-old who has had difficulty swallowing over the last 3 months.

1. **Food.** Initially only food stuck (meat and apples particularly). This has become progressively worse so that now even soft foods, such as stewed fruit and bread, stick. Initially there was some pain when it stuck, but none recently. It seemed to stick a few seconds after being swallowed rather than being regurgitated immediately.

2. **Liquids.** For the last 3 weeks you have noticed difficulty with liquids as well.

3. **Cough.** 3 days ago you began to cough violently a few seconds after taking food or fluids, and have become short of breadth.

4. **Weight loss.** You have lost 2 stones in weight over the last 6–8 months, and are still losing weight.

5. **Past medical/social history.** Minor heartburn in past (self-treated with milk and antacids); no previous difficulty swallowing. Smokes 20/day, drinks 10 pints/week. Married. Job: teacher.

Box 26.3   OSCE station on dysphagia: examiner's sheet

Dysphagia station: examiner's sheet

Student name _____ Exam number _____

One mark to be given for general enquiry in area concerned, two marks for further enquiry or exploration.

(Note to examiner: remind student to suggest investigations and diagnosis if required.)

Duration of symptoms	2	1	0
Immediate regurgitation/coughing	2	1	0
Progression of dysphagia	2	1	0
Dysphagia solids and/or liquids	2	1	0
Time after swallowing that things stick	2	1	0
Impact pain on swallowing: time course	2	1	0
Weight loss: time course	2	1	0
PMH (previous medical history) of heartburn/regurgitation	2	1	0
Social history (smoking/alcohol)	2	1	0
Develops cough after a few seconds	2	1	0
Provisional diagnosis of (advanced) carcinoma	2	1	0
Additional diagnosis of possible fistula (max. 1 mark)		1	0
Two investigations to help confirm diagnosis	2	1	0
(Chest X-ray, CT scan, contrast swallow, endoscopy, not FBC (full blood count), etc.)			

Examiner's initials _____ Total score (max 25) _____

Communication skills:

Please circle **one** *number to indicate your level of agreement with this statement:* 'Student's general approach and communication skills are satisfactory for this stage of his/her career'

Strongly agree   [5]   [4]   [3]   [2]   [1]   Strongly disagree the examiner is also given (Box 26.3). This covers the areas that the designers of the station thought it important for the student to consider. Note the section at the end, which considers the student's communication skills and approach to the patient. The examiner also has a copy of the instructions to the student and the 'patient'.

Most students prefer the OSCE style of exam to the traditional format because it is seen as fair in that it samples plenty of areas of skills and knowledge. You are not likely to be caught out by a selection of 'unlucky' and unfamiliar topics. The thoughtful student also appreciates other things. First, there is a limit to the variety of things that can be tested in a 6-minute station. Second, OSCE marking schemes take a lot of time and effort to put together, so they are likely to be used more than once. Ask last year's students what came up. This is not strange advice to come from an examiner. I am concerned that my students should reach a set standard. If knowing that they will probably have stations on examining the fundus or basic life support means they will learn these techniques, that is fine by me. I want to encourage competence. Increasingly, exams are being seen as a means of promoting flow and not as a filtration mechanism.

27

Revision and exams

'Examinations are not a matter of life or death, they're much more important than that.'

This view is one that many students would echo, and though it is several years since I last sat an exam even writing about them now speeds my pulse and makes my mouth go slightly dry. If exams are so important, why is this one of the shorter chapters of this book? The answer is simple. If you have read and taken notice of the rest of the book, you will have learnt patterns of study which will ensure that you will pass the exams. The sections on good writing, MCQs, clinical work and planning your time all provide guidance in specific areas. Much of the following has already been considered or implied.

Let us re-emphasize some points. We do not fail a set percentage of students. If you are good enough to pass, you will be passed. In fact only a small percentage of students fail and if you follow the advice in this book you will not be among them. The questions we set are searching of your knowledge and understanding, but they are not 'trick' questions.

REVISION

The key to successful revision is to start in adequate time, plan carefully and think about what you are trying to do. Starting in adequate time means planning a timetable which anticipates having completed everything 3 or 4 days before the exam date. This leaves you with time to cope with the unexpected. *Plan your time and plan your method.* Planning your time means writing out a realistic timetable covering all the topics that you need to revise. Do you cover something once or several times? You will remember and understand more of a topic if you cover it three times in separate slots to a total of 3 hours over a fortnight than you will by spending 3 hours at one sitting. *Remember: spaced learning promotes retention and recall.* Planning your time also means building in flexibility and breaks. As well as planning your time, you will want to plan your method. If you have taken any notice of the earlier chapters, your notes will in the main be reasonably organized and summarized. If not, that is your first task. Methods will vary but many find it useful to summarize and condense topics progressively until each can be fitted into a postcard-sized space filled with main headings and subheadings on one side and simple diagrams, brief notes and links with other areas and cards on the other. These cards form a portable revision pack, for use in bus queues etc. as well as at more formal revision times. Whatever method you choose, make sure that it is active and involves more than just staring at notes or a textbook.

Use available information sources. Does the library or department have any old exam papers? Can your tutors tell you what sorts of topic are likely to come up? If you have no joy from these two sources, then ask last year's students what topics they were asked about. They may or may not be asked again in your exam but they will give you practice at writing answers. All that is honest is fair in revising for exams. Working in pairs or small groups for some of the time can save a lot of work. Swop and discuss outline answers to past questions, explain topics to each other and let each write outline answers to the same questions. How does your approach and coverage differ from your friend's? Try a few full answers under exam conditions and time constraints. Evaluate your answers and their structure with reference to the advice given in the 'Good writing' chapter of this guide. With practice, and working with someone you trust, you can quickly become good at objectively assessing the quality of each other's work.

The following two exercises are quite fun, and very illuminating for a small group. Take a topic. Another group member chooses your SOLO level. Each member sketches out an outline answer at a standard such that it would meet one of the five levels of the SOLO taxonomy (see Chapter 12). Defend the reasons why your answer meets its required SOLO level – no lower and no higher. Look back at a few of your other answers to past questions. Which SOLO level do they meet? The second exercise involves taking a pair of topics, which you judge you can write about equally well. Under exam conditions (say, 30 minutes per question) write out answers for each. There is an additional rule. For one answer, you *must* start writing the answer within 30 seconds. For the other answer, you are *not allowed* to write any of the essay for the first 5 minutes – only to plan the outline. Imagine you are marking. Which produced the better answer?

PROJECT WORK AND LABORATORY WORK

A reminder. These may form a separate part of your assessed work. Ask your tutors whether this is so, and if so what proportion of your overall mark they constitute. *Note also that attendance at these sessions may be a requirement for you to continue on the course, even if they are not formally assessed or they carry only a small number of marks.* Do not ignore practical work in your revision because exam questions may well be based on knowledge derived from it even if, for instance, the laboratory workbooks are not taken in and marked.

THE EXAM

Be well-prepared and well-rested, having taken some time off to relax the day before and to have an early night. You will arrive at the exam room in good time and will find someone to talk to about topics other than the exam. Now is not the time for attempting last-minute revision. If you have planned your studies and revision using the advice in this guide, you will have the knowledge to pass the exam. Think positive. You will be nervous. So will all those around you. Continue to think positive, take a few deep breaths and concentrate on relaxing groups of muscles which are tense. *Mild* controlled anxiety will enhance your performance, not detract from it.

So, you are prepared and will pass. What can make the well-prepared candidate fail a written exam? Three things. Not reading the instructions, not answering the questions and not keeping to time. Little else.

Read the instructions carefully and underline the key words. *'Answer **three** questions, **one** from each section'* means just that. Not 'answer all the questions' or 'any three'. Read through each question. Turn over the exam paper to check whether there are questions or sections on the back as well. Decide which you are going to tackle, if you have a choice. If not, then choose a question you feel you can answer well. Read through it and underline key phrases: <u>analyze</u>, <u>compare</u> and <u>contrast,</u> <u>list</u> the features of, write <u>short notes</u> on <u>three</u> of the following. On exam papers, words retain their normal English meaning: 'analyze' does not suddenly mean 'list', nor does 'short notes' mean 'write a four-page essay'!

Write an outline of the answer first, as you have practised during revision. For a 25-minute answer use 5 minutes for this. Write a structured answer, as discussed earlier in this guide. Make sure that your writing remains legible. Always plan your time and keep to it. Check the length of the exam. Ninety minutes for three questions means 25 minutes per question, 10 minutes to check through at the end and 5 minutes to read right through the paper at the start. Marks are easy to pick up at the start of an essay, and become progressively more difficult to earn. You will do better by achieving, say, 60%, 56%, 58% than by splitting your time poorly and getting 75%, 55%, 10%.

MCQs are rather different. You must of course read the instructions and each question carefully, but as previously noted generally all questions are to be attempted. Start at the beginning and work your way through. If there is a question you find confusing then mark it in the margin and come back to it. Watch the time. As discussed before, if there is a negative marking system you should not guess. If there is neutral marking you must attempt everything. Make sure you know the marking system before you sit the exam.

After the exam there is the tense wait for the results. When you get them, that should not be the end. Try to get some feedback on your performance which will help you next time. Think back as to whether there was any area that seemed particularly hard, and try to work out why and what you can do about it. If you have severe difficulties, discuss them with your tutor or the Academic Sub-Dean. If you just pass, don't overdo the sackcloth and ashes; not everyone is in the top 10%, and those who are do not always make the best clinicians.

If it is Finals and you pass, just celebrate. Forget your ranking – everyone else will.

28

Moving on: PRHO year and beyond

You're qualified. Done the ceremony, got the certificate, had the congratulations, back-slapped and/or kissed your colleagues. Felt that sense of pride at the first batch of envelopes correctly giving you the title 'Dr' before your name. No matter that they are mostly from insurance companies, offering a loan or advertising a car appropriate to your new-found status. Looking at the envelopes still makes you feel great. And so it should. To qualify as a doctor is a tremendous achievement.

Now for the next stage, the PRHO (Pre-Registration House Officer) year. The transition used to be tough and rough. Now, increasingly, it is smooth but still huge. The improvement is due largely to the work of the GMC and postgraduate deans. Recommendations for general clinical training, which forms the final year of basic medical training (the preregistration year), are contained in the booklet *The New Doctor*, published by the GMC in 1997. You should have been given a copy; if not, approach your medical school or postgraduate dean.

This chapter looks at the structure of the PRHO year and what you can expect from it; what the responsibilities of others are towards you; and what your responsibilities are to yourself, patients and colleagues. It will also briefly look beyond.

You will work as a PRHO for 12 months before full registration. There are three basic patterns of work:

- 6 months' surgery/6 months' medicine
- 4 months' surgery/4 months' medicine/4 months' another specialty (including GP)
- 3 months' surgery/3 months' surgical specialty/3 months' medicine/3 months' medical specialty.

The order of posts within these patterns will vary. The first of the three patterns is by far the most common. The posts may be in a hospital or a health centre – again, the first is by far the most common. Posts in health centres have been limited by several requirements, one being that the health centre has had to have a close working relationship with the university's general practice department or unit. Until recently, to satisfy Section 12 of the Medical Act 1983, health centres accommodating PRHO posts had to be located in 'publicly-owned premises'. This was a historical anomaly because now, unlike in 1983, few health centres are within the public domain, being financed and owned by the GPs rather than rented. These premises are often superbly designed, equipped and organized. There is no obvious or logical reason why many of these health centres could not provide suitable posts just because they are not 'publicly owned', and Section 12 of the Medical Act 1983 has now been updated.

Posts of less than 3 months' duration are generally not approved as part of PRHO training. This is because it takes time to build relationships within the working environment so that you can profit from the experience available, and less than 3 months is too short. A note of caution. Look carefully at the structure of PRHO posts for which you apply. A 6-month rotation around, say, three medical consultants may be couched in terms of 'providing broader experience' but can mean that you never have time to get really involved as part of a single team. Similarly, if the PRHOs are ward-based rather than consultant-based talk to the current post-holders about the exact meaning of 'ward-based', how well they know all the consultants whose patients they look after and how well those consultants know them.

Which pattern should you go for? In truth it matters little – it is not the pattern but the clinical experience and training that you get within the posts that makes a rotation good or bad. How do you decide? The surest way is simple. Ask a current or recent incumbent if he/she would recommend the post to a friend. If the answer is 'Yes' you are probably on to a winner. The other way to get to know what a post is like is to act as a shadow to the house officer for a few weeks during your final year. This is being strongly encouraged by the GMC. The problem is that by the time you shadow you will usually already be committed to the post, and so you may gain forewarning without remedy. However, due to the activity of postgraduate deans there are far, far fewer poor posts than there were even 5 years ago.

If you are thinking about general practice, but are unsure, there is an argument for taking a rotation which includes general practice. If you are determined to stay in hospital practice there is perhaps an even stronger argument for spending a few months in general practice so that you have some knowledge of what the 'real world', as GPs often refer to it, is like.

What you can expect from your training is laid out by the GMC in *The New Doctor*. The GMC expects that all PRHOs be provided with high quality education and training, and that those who supply this should themselves be trained in educational supervision. The responsibility for ensuring that training takes place rests with the universities, postgraduate deans, clinical tutors and the PRHO's educational supervisors. PRHOs also have responsibility for their own education, and must be prepared to demonstrate that they have made sufficient progress during the year to achieve full registration. Progress includes not only a developed knowledge base and skills base but also the adoption of the GMC's guidance as detailed in its publication *Good Medical Practice*. One peculiarity is that while you are still partly the responsibility of the university during the year, I do not believe that the university receives any fee for you.

As a PRHO you are learning to become a doctor partly by providing a service. As acknowledgement of this service commitment you will receive a salary which is approximately the average for a full-time male worker. Not negligible. Your practice must be supervised, and there must always be someone of a higher grade available *within the hospital* to whom you can turn. Your workload must be 'reasonable', and this should take into account not only the number of patients you look after but also their distribution within the hospital and the nature of their problems. Every job has a quota of routine tasks, but certain tasks are not the responsibility of the PRHO and some will generally be undertaken by others but sometimes by the PRHO. The former group includes filing (as opposed to checking) path reports, finding beds and transporting blood samples or request cards. The latter group includes routine phlebotomy and the clerking of multiple day-cases undergoing routine diagnostic and therapeutic procedures. The number of hours you work, and the intensity of your on-call commitments, is regulated by the 'New Deal' arrangements. If a post requires doctors to work for more than the set number of hours on a regular basis, it will cease to be recognized as a PRHO post. We are of course professionals and at times we work extra hours to ensure the welfare of our patients, who are always out first concern.

You will be supervised by more senior staff, who will include a named consultant. You will also have a named educational supervisor. These two may be, and often are, the same person. During each PRHO post, time must be set aside for discussion of your progress and to look at the training opportunities that the post offers. There is a move towards the use of logbooks and records of clinical training to help form a basis for these discussions.

As well as clinical training, a controlled workload and structured supervision can you expect anything more? You can expect reasonable quality, clean accommodation and catering arrangements which take into account that you work throughout the 24 hours. Unchanged bed-linen and a plate of curling sandwiches are not acceptable.

As well as ensuring that PRHOs are adequately supervised, the GMC and postgraduate deans have insisted that there is a mandatory induction period. This covers important areas, including those of a medico-legal nature (e.g. handling of complaints, death certification) and the practices and procedures of the trust for which you are to work. Many trusts supply a house officers' handbook, which contains much practical information such as information about resuscitation training, and guidelines for the therapy and management of common clinical conditions. If such a handbook is to be provided, request it a few weeks before you start. You will be so busy at the start of your job that otherwise it is unlikely to be read but used only as an emergency reference guide.

A handover between old and new PRHO is encouraged to help ensure clinical continuity, although that responsibility falls to all members of the clinical team. This handover is easier to arrange for the first house job (generally in August) than the second, when both old and new are changing post. It falls apart when the house officer takes the last 2 weeks of the job off as annual leave, a common and understandable practice. During your final year as a student you may have the opportunity to shadow the house officer in the post and hospital where you will be doing your first house job. You get to know the layout of the hospital, who is who and how routine things are organized. This means that your first few weeks as a house officer will be far less fraught than otherwise and, if available, it is an opportunity well worth taking. If not offered, seek permission to do it for a few weeks in the final year in place of something else. You may not succeed but if student demand is generated, and the GMC wish it, pressure to change the system for subsequent years can be considerable. Altruism gives the heart a warm glow.

Despite induction and improved supervision, which have smoothed the transition, there is no doubt that becoming a PRHO is associated with a steep learning curve. The difference between the new graduate and those 3 months into the PRHO year is usually immense, so don't expect too much of yourself immediately. Your more senior colleagues expect and are expected to provide support. Remember, at the corresponding time next year you will be providing support to a PRHO of the next generation.

During the second half of the PRHO year you should receive careers advice if required. It may be that you are undecided on your final choice of specialty or you need guidance as to what jobs to apply for in your chosen specialty. Many will have decided their path. If you have not, my advice would be to take your time. You could be practising medicine for 40 years. The postgraduate dean, or a person designated by the dean, will provide advice but often those already working in the specialty can provide the most relevant information. If you really wish to practise a specialty such as gastroenterology, radiology or anaesthetics, be neither unduly encouraged nor discouraged by people telling you it is a shortage or glut specialty. During the time it takes to undergo further specialist training, the situation may well change.

In all specialties you will meet the contented and the discontented. Whichever specialty you choose, it will provide opportunities for challenge and interest. Whether you are happy and fulfilled depends not on the specialty itself but on your compatibility with it and the conditions of the actual post you hold. It also depends on achieving a balance between your professional working life and your personal life. The balance point varies from person to person and may vary also at different times in your career. It is something that you have to decide for yourself. One person may choose a direct path to achieve a consultant post or general practice position with the minimum of delay. Another may wish for time out or part-time work in order to go abroad, be involved in bringing up a family or for other reasons. Seek advice about which options will smooth or hinder your career path. But in the end make sure that you choose the path which will meet *your definition* of personal success and fulfilment, not those of others. The smoothest and straightest path does not always provide the best view.

By the time that you have completed a *Tomorrow's Doctors* medical course and *New Doctor* PRHO training and of course read this book, you will not only be an established professional but also have all the skills and abilities required to ensure you can keep up to date throughout your professional life.

Being a doctor is a privilege and an honour. Congratulations to you on deciding that it is to be your choice of career.

References

References

General Medical Council 1993 Tomorrow's doctors. Recommendations on Undergraduate Medical Education

General Medical Council 1995 Good medical practice

General Medical Council 1997 The new doctor

Rowntree D 1998 Learn to study, 4th edn. (Warner, London)

Index